A Navy Nurse's Memoir of Healthcare Transformation

A Navy Nurse's Memoir of Healthcare Transformation

Unlocking Innovation: Harnessing Personal and Professional Insights to Revolutionize Healthcare with Virtual Reality

From Sea Stories to Virtual Realities

CDR (Ret) Dagoberto Salinas Jr., MSN, RN, ACCNS-AG, CNOR, VA-BC, NC, USN

Published by Game Changer Publishing

Paperback ISBN: 978-1-964811-69-7
Hardcover ISBN: 978-1-964811-08-6
Digital ISBN: 978-1-964811-09-3

NOTE: Numbers appearing in superscript, such as [1], indicate a citation found in the "References" section at the end of the book.

IMAGES NOTE: The appearance of U.S. Department of Defense (DoD) visual information does not imply or constitute DoD endorsement.

GC GAME CHANGER PUBLISHING
www.GameChangerPublishing.com

Dedication

To my wife, Scarlet, for restoring my desire to live again.

"Ask and it will be given to you; seek and you will find; knock and the door will be opened to you. For everyone who asks receives; the one who seeks finds; and to the one who knocks, the door will be opened."

Matthew 7:7-8

A Navy Nurse's Memoir of Healthcare Transformation

Unlocking Innovation: Harnessing Personal and Professional Insights to Revolutionize Healthcare with Virtual Reality

From Sea Stories to Virtual Realities

Dagoberto Salinas Jr.

GAME CHANGER PUBLISHING

www.GameChangerPublishing.com

Foreword

I first ran into the name of Dagoberto Salinas when I was a seasoned U.S. Navy Sailor enjoying myself back at my hometown in South Texas as your friendly neighborhood recruiter following two Western Pacific deployments aboard one of the Navy's finest destroyers—USS Harry W. Hill (DD-986). I was a hardened and experienced sailor with years of experience operating in the harshest environments. On a combat ship, operations at sea are the closest most people will ever know to the "razor's edge," rough sea climate under the most extreme weather conditions, constantly aware that the ocean is unforgiving. I had seen and learned a thing or two, so not too many people impressed me. Then came future Commander (CDR) Salinas, a high school senior at J.W. Nixon HS in Laredo, TX.

During one of my recruiting cold calls, Dago accepted the offer to learn more about the Navy. His high school academic record was impeccable, and his extracurricular activities were commendable. I knew he was a young man (17 years of age) with unlimited potential, so it placed me and the other two seasoned sailors in the office in what I could only describe as a high-stakes, high-pressure environment where our split-second decisions could change one's life forever. It was our Navy "NFL draft" day when you took your pick. I will admit that I was impressed. On paper, Dago was competitive enough to gain admission to any top 4-year academic institution in the U.S., but his family's financial constraints would make that option extremely difficult. Instead, he chose the Navy, knowing that he would eventually achieve his goal of becoming a healthcare professional. I was blessed to become a part of his journey—from his early days at sea as an enlisted member to his commission as a naval officer. I was there at the beginning of his naval career as he shipped off to boot camp, and I was there 23 years later to welcome him back home at his retirement celebration alongside his family in Laredo.

Dago spent his formidable naval career fine-tuning his gifts—his intelligence, discipline, and perseverance. Over the years, he has sacrificed his time caring for patients at home and abroad, and his impact is recognized globally. After reading this book, it's evident that his resolve to influence others has remained intact. He seeks to encompass his highly-tuned skill sets through the modern era of technology. Better yet, he's committed to transforming the healthcare education and training landscape. The ever-changing nature of our healthcare system calls for a change, and Dago is at the forefront of it all. Knowing who he is and where he came from (which you will soon learn through this book), I know he will continue to make a difference.

Welcome aboard.

CWO (Ret) Ignacio Garza, USN

Table of Contents

Introduction

If you know me well, you are probably wondering, *What in the world does Dago have to write about?* I asked myself the same question. But, if you don't know me well, you will most likely decide whether or not to read this book within the next few seconds; it will appeal most to healthcare innovators, educators, students, clinicians, administrators, military service members, or veterans, and even entrepreneurs because, as the title implies, it is about harnessing personal and professional insights to revolutionize education and training practices in healthcare. In my case, the insights were drawn from my military service. I hope that it will also encourage you, the reader, to reflect on your life experiences and leverage them to make the world a better place.

I had no reason to write other than to share a recent epiphany about using VR technology to improve how vascular access specialists are educated and trained. But that same idea evolved into thinking: "What the heck? Why not use VR as an adjunct to enhance the learning experience in healthcare everywhere? I felt the need to put it all in writing since it's the best way to express my thoughts—I can't picture myself doing webinars, podcasting, YouTubing, etc.

I believe that it is no coincidence that you are where you are today. Every step that you have taken, good or bad, has led you to make certain decisions. These life experiences influence what you do today and what you will eventually do tomorrow. Decisions to study in a particular field, work in a specific industry, get married and start a family, buy a home, make calculated investments, or start a business: make them all count.

This book will take you through my journey—pre- and post-military, as well as my experience while on active duty—and give you a glimpse into how and why I founded a VR implementation consulting company called CLINSPEC Solutions, LLC. I will share examples of how immersive VR can enhance traditional education and training modalities in healthcare. If you are a healthcare stakeholder, I challenge you to explore these innovative solutions further and contemplate adopting them to augment your existing practices. My uncle—Ray Quiñones, a retired United States Army lieutenant colonel—once told me that planning missions was the easiest part of his job, but executing them was the hardest. As such, I will also delve into considerations for VR implementation and sustainment to help alleviate some of the fears many associate with change of this caliber. There are many different models to choose from, but I will share my preferred methods for structuring your implementation approach through real-life examples.

You will see me reference the movie *Forrest Gump* (my all-time favorite movie) a few times throughout the book, but the stories and names of people, places, and organizations are all real. There are some people that I purposefully omitted from the core content because adding them would have added extra chapters. Instead, I will give them credit right here at the start. I refer to the multi-service unit (MSU) civilian staff who served at Naval Hospital Jacksonville between 2016 and 2019. Thank you for restoring me personally and professionally as I entered this command after facing personal obstacles. During this period, I discovered my true strengths and weaknesses and fully committed myself to shaping healthcare practices at the highest level. The civilian registered nurses (RNs) in the MSU were my biggest supporters and critics. Their feedback was always honest, and they were not afraid to speak up. This is exactly how leaders are developed, and I will forever be grateful for their support.

Each chapter is presented chronologically, from my middle school years to the present (June 2024). As you read through them, consider your own education and training environments and ask yourself the following three questions.

1. What were the most challenging aspects of these environments?
2. How were these challenges commonly addressed?
3. Can VR offer solutions to these challenges?

At the end of chapters 3-8, I will share examples of VR solutions and supporting evidence to enlighten you on what education researchers have been working on. I challenge you to reflect on your own personal and professional experiences and put your ideas into action:

Put It Into Action

Chapter #	Topics/themes
3	Healthcare Communications and Undergraduate Nursing Education
4	Nursing skills, Perioperative Nursing, Empathy Development, and NICU Nursing
5	Cultural Competency, Teamwork and Safety, and Combat Casualty Care
6	Surgical Education, Trauma Care, Critical Care, and Laboratory Environment
7	Vascular Access and Grand Rounds
8	Anatomy Education, Basic Life Support, and Pre-hospital Training

Most of the examples I'll provide center on healthcare, but keep an open mind to VR and how it could be applied to training in other industries like construction, transportation, agriculture, retail, food and beverage, and more.

The possibilities are endless. The first time I ever donned a VR headset, I dropped one of the hand controls on the floor because it felt like I was placing it on a real table in front of me. That's exactly what training should feel like—as real as possible!

Long ago, when I first met my book writer friend John P. Roach Jr. in San Diego, California, I knew I would write a book someday; I just didn't know when. If writing a book is on your mind, or you strongly believe in accomplishing something, do it! I dedicated three solid months to writing, translating to approximately 450 words per day, seven days per week. If you think about it, it's almost like writing a college essay every day for three months straight. It is not as bad as it sounds, but it is a sacrifice—one that is worth every keystroke. If you decide to write your own story, start by going on a long walk and brainstorm ideas. Then, find some quiet time (for me, it was at five in the morning in my home garage) and play some music to get your neurons fired up. It may sound odd, but the sound of Claude Debussy's music gets me to write as much as the *Rocky IV* soundtrack makes me want to work out and say, "No pain, no gain." Just pace yourself as if you were planning to run a full marathon.

I hope you enjoy the read. From the bottom of my heart, thank you for being part of my journey!

CHAPTER 1

Let the Journey Begin

My interest in the health professions began while I was in middle school. It was at Secundaria Num. 4 Reforma in Monterrey, Mexico, that I was first exposed to real science. We didn't just read about science; we lived it. We learned to observe, ask questions, hypothesize, experiment, evaluate results, and make conclusions based on results. From dissecting insects to molding glass rods over open flames to donating our own sperm to examine flagella under a microscope, we did it all. Our scientific projects brought science to life. However, the pressure of identifying a career at that age was also very real. Professional studies in Mexico and many other countries begin right after high school, and one must decide whether to pursue a trade job or a professional career as early as middle school. Considering my strong interest in anatomy and physiology, genetics, chemistry, and general biology, everything pointed toward a career in the medical field.

In 1992, my family and I moved to Monterrey from my birthplace of Houston, Texas, due to my father's work. At the time, my dad was working for a transportation company called Consolidated FreightWays (CF). CF had offered him a promotion as a regional sales manager in northern Mexico (most of our family still lived in Mexico, while some had decided to migrate to Houston in the late 1970s). Living in Monterrey accelerated my maturity level as a young kid, and it wasn't by choice. I might have matured quicker than usual because the public school I initially enrolled in, Dr. Ignacio Morones Prieto, made an administrative error that resulted in me skipping fourth grade—from third straight into fifth grade. The curriculum was so advanced that I didn't have time to play games. I feared failing a grade, so I buckled myself down in hopes of catching up with my peers.

Worse, I didn't know how to read or write in Spanish! I give my aunt Elisa Cavazos all the credit for tutoring me every day after school in fifth grade to help me learn the basics. Mexico was also one of those places where you either stood up for yourself or fell victim to bullying. So, I learned how to fight and study.

A career in transportation, however, often leads to a nomadic lifestyle. In my last year of middle school, 1995, my father again accepted another work transfer, this time to Laredo, Texas, where I enrolled at Laredo Christian Academy.

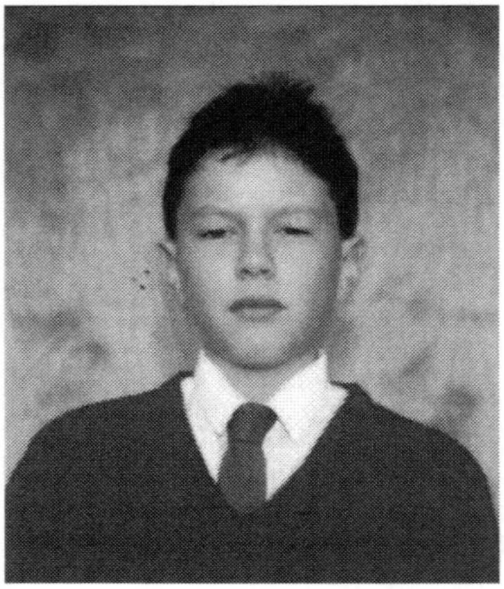

There is a common saying in Spanish: "*el perico verde donde quiera es verde.*" This translates to "a green parakeet remains green no matter where it goes." As I transitioned back to the United States, I excelled in my science courses thanks to the rigorous studies I had completed in Mexico. I also brought with me the dream of someday becoming a physician. Keeping my dream alive was not the problem; the challenge was that I moved from one school to another due to my father's job, and career guidance wasn't as readily accessible as it is now via the internet. Only a year after moving to Laredo, we moved to Chula Vista, California.

My first week in California, I found myself walking the halls of Chula Vista High School and getting approached by a cholo who sported a shaved head and a "wife beater," and baggy pants. We made eye contact, and the cholo said, "What up, dawg?" Not knowing the California lingo, I thought the cholo had said, "What up, *dago*?" I immediately thought that this was such a friendly place. What a naïve teen I was! It was at Chula Vista HS where I learned physical and mental strength through athletics, specifically wrestling and cross-country.

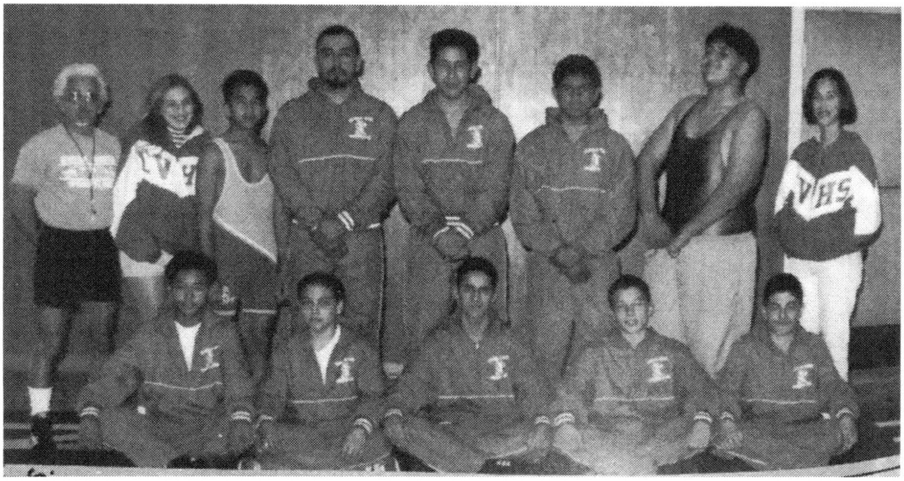

Only a year later, my family returned to Laredo, TX, where I continued my high school studies at J.W. Nixon High School. As a junior at J.W. Nixon HS, I decided to get a head start in college by accepting an opportunity to join the school's inaugural concurrent enrollment program at Texas A&M International University in 1997. I was ready to begin pursuing a medical profession, but finances at home were not looking too good. I vividly remember the day I asked my mom for $50 to pay the concurrent enrollment fee. Sadly, my mother looked at me and said we didn't have enough funds to cover the cost.

So, I returned to school the next day to tell my HS counselor that I would have to respectfully decline the opportunity because we didn't have the money to pay the fee. I will never forget the moment that Mrs. Navarro reached into her purse, took the amount out of her own wallet, and said, "Here, *mijo*. You can't let this opportunity pass. I know that you will someday return to pay it back." This kind gesture made me shed some tears in her office, and I vowed to pay her back (I returned two years later to double the amount she had given me as a show of gratitude). But at that moment, I realized that attending college was going to be more challenging than I thought and that I would need a solid plan.

One day, while walking around Mall del Norte— what teens in Laredo did for fun—I saw an Army soldier talking with another youngster inside a military recruiting office. I also noticed several high-tech posters advertising recruitment and money for college, so I thought that maybe I, too, should visit one of the recruiting offices—all of the military branches had one in the mall—to get more information. I remember entering the Army's recruiting office and seeing posters of helicopters, weapons, parachutes, tanks, and one of a healthcare provider (clean-shaven, smiling, and with a stethoscope around his neck). I thought, hey, maybe I could become an army physician.

The stern voice of a recruiter snapped me out of my musings. "Hey, what can I do for you?"

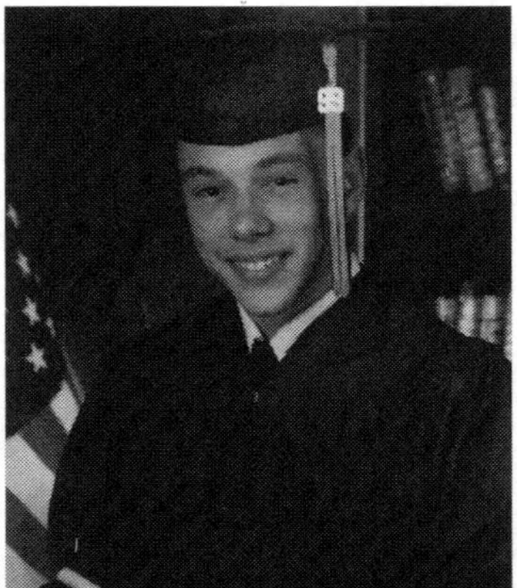

I said, "Just checking to see if you offer any college programs. I am interested in the medical field."

"How old are you?" he asked. When I told him I was sixteen, he said, "*Nombre vato*, do me a favor. Put your name on this roster. I will add you into our system and give you a call when you turn seventeen."

I left a bit disillusioned, but at least I had discovered that the military was an option.

A year later, a navy recruiter named Torpedoman's Mate 2nd Class Ignacio Garza called my home. He asked, "Have you ever considered joining the Navy to travel the world?" I said that I hadn't, but I was open to learning more about it. Although I was still only seventeen years old, he said they could still get me to join with my parent's permission. Of course, I asked about college and the chances of becoming a

Navy physician, and when I confirmed my 4.0 GPA, he assured me that it was very possible. The rest is history. On July 19, 1999, I said goodbye to my parents, my younger sister Stephany (July 19 was her 10th birthday), my grandmother Dora, my aunt Magda, my cousin "Machu," and her husband Humberto at Mall del Norte.

I didn't want my family to see my tears rolling down my cheeks (I also had a knot in my throat), so once I turned away, I never looked back. I was excited about this new adventure but sad to leave my family. I knew that it was time to fulfill the dream I had envisioned a few years ago while in middle school. A few hours later, I was on a Greyhound bus headed northbound on I-35 for final processing at the Military Entrance Processing Station (MEPS) in San Antonio, Texas.

My first night away from home was a bit surreal. About a dozen other navy recruits were lingering in the Knights Inn parking lot, and they were also awaiting final processing and shipment to basic training in Great Lakes, Illinois (or "Great Mistakes," as we later learned to call it). Back then, there were no cell phones to distract us, so we mingled, forming bonds and sharing our backgrounds. I remember meeting a recruit who said he was rated as a hospital corpsman (HM) and would be receiving his training at Great Lakes Naval Hospital Corps School (HM "A" School). As a point of reference, technical schools in the Navy are known as "A" schools, and jobs are known as rates.

Reminiscing a year before that moment in the Knight's Inn parking lot, the recruiter at MEPS had also reassured me that I could go to HM "A" School. However, I would later learn that there was a huge caveat to that statement. When I first met with the MEPS recruiter, whose job is to help you find a military job based on your qualifying Armed Services Vocational Aptitude Battery (ASVAB) scores, he reiterated that the HM rate was "packed" and that I would have to wait another year to ship out if that was the path I wanted to take. My ASVAB scores were higher than average, and there were incentives to choose other rates, but I was fixated on the opportunity to work in the medical field. I was not too fond of waiting around in Laredo for another year, so I opened myself up to other options that would eventually lead to me becoming an HM.

After declining other options, the MEPS recruiter introduced me to a "special" program called Seaman Apprenticeship. Through it, I would get the opportunity to explore different rates by shadowing and then selecting my rate of choice. When I asked how long the process was, the recruiter said it would only take three weeks of post-boot camp training at Naval Training Center (NTC) in Great Lakes. I figured three weeks of extra training was worth the opportunity, so I signed the contract.

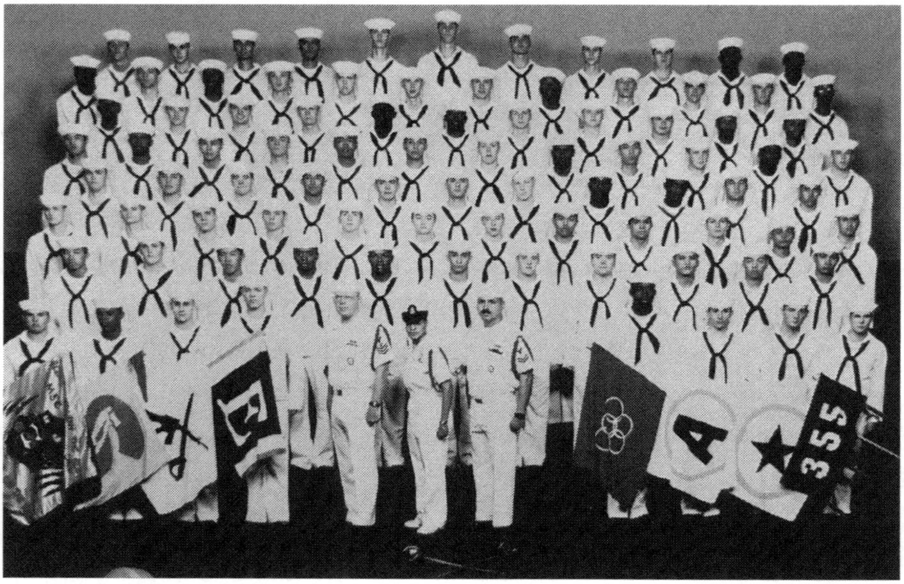

The ten-week boot camp experience was interesting. I regretted signing up on day one; it got easier toward the middle, and by the last day, I just wanted to get out of there. The one thing I eventually appreciated about boot camp was discovering that humans can practically learn anything through repetitive practice. If you think about it, boot camp is full of recruits from all over the country. In a short period, they learn how to make their racks, shine their boots, prepare for inspections, iron their uniforms, properly wear the uniform, march synchronously, work as a team, and follow instructions carefully. Recruits deliberately practice over and over until they get it right.

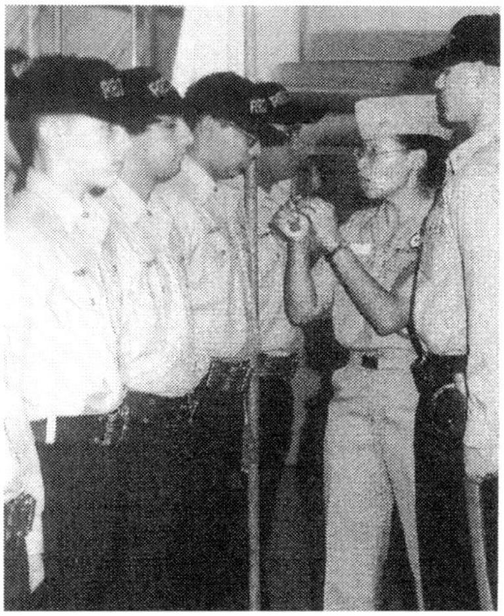

One major event that all recruits practice for, regardless of which military branch they serve under, is what is known as "pass in review." It's a tradition where a high-ranking officer reviews the readiness of military recruits before graduation. It's a pretty big deal, so it must be done perfectly. To help make sure this happened and to make it feel real for everyone beforehand, it was important to practice where the actual pass in review was to take place. The main takeaway in basic training was that success was determined by how and where we practiced. Training in a realistic environment was key, whether it was learning how to march, put out a ship fire, or respond to medical emergencies. The concept of "training like you fight" was ingrained in me from the start of my naval career.

My last day of boot camp was one of the worst days I experienced during the training. We had been granted a day of liberty after completing our pass in review and were given clear instructions on how to dress and when to return to the barracks (we actually called them ships). Unfortunately, one of our fellow recruits broke curfew, which also got the rest of us in trouble. We were all supposed to look after each other, but we failed. Consequently, our recruit division commander suspended our transfer out of boot camp until further notice. Spending more time there and delaying our training orders sounded horrible. My only comfort that day was seeing my family once more.

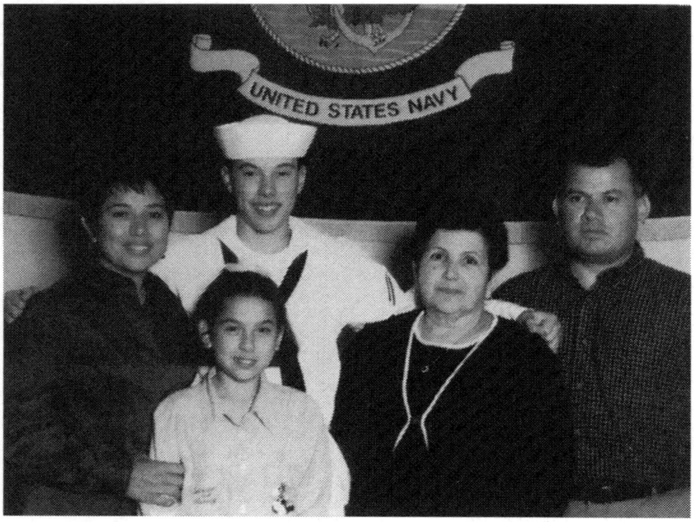

Shortly after the suspension was lifted, I relocated to Surface Warfare Training Command (literally next door to Recruit Training Command), where many new sailors begin their skills training. It was the end of September 1999, and it was already too cold for me. I vividly remember sporting my new uniform peacoat and sticking my cold, numb hands in my warm pockets. Within a minute of doing so, I heard someone yell, "Get your hands out of your pockets!" It was muffled due to the distance from which it came, so I looked at my buddies—Adrian Arriola from El Paso, Texas, and Angel Treviño from San Antonio—and asked, "What is this guy saying?" None of us could tell. Then it came again, clearer this time, and I learned that, apparently, uniform pockets were not intended to be used as pockets.

At this point, I still didn't know my fate, and I had no idea that my understanding of the seaman apprenticeship program was off. The MEPS recruiter in San Antonio didn't lie about me having to attend a three-week training program after boot camp, but didn't disclose how long it would take me to make it to HM "A" School after the apprenticeship program. Apparently, the minimum requirement was to serve two years aboard a naval ship as an undesignated deck seaman. There was only one way to get out of this service requirement: score the highest GPA in my seaman apprenticeship class. I had good study habits, so I knew this would be possible. My biggest competitor was Seaman Craig B. Wibberley, but rather than compete against each other, we studied together. I can't remember what rate he was pursuing, but it was clear that his ambitions were as strong as mine.

Ultimately, we tied for 1st place in a class of about forty sailors. We were excited to know we had qualified to skip the undesignated seaman service requirement and go straight to "A" school. All we needed was the official message. On the second to last day in the program, however, our chief petty officer walked into our class to officially deliver what we thought would be good news (SN Wibberley and I nodded at each other as a sign of "Yeah, we made it!") Instead, we were informed that the computer system that allowed them to redesignate sailors had crashed. They had no timeline for fixing it, so we would all have to go to the fleet to serve our respective times. We were devastated to hear the news but somewhat relieved that at least we would be going to familiar places. I received orders to serve aboard USS Valley Forge (CG-50), a guided-missile cruiser based out of San Diego that sported the motto, "FIRST IN WAR - FIRST IN PEACE."

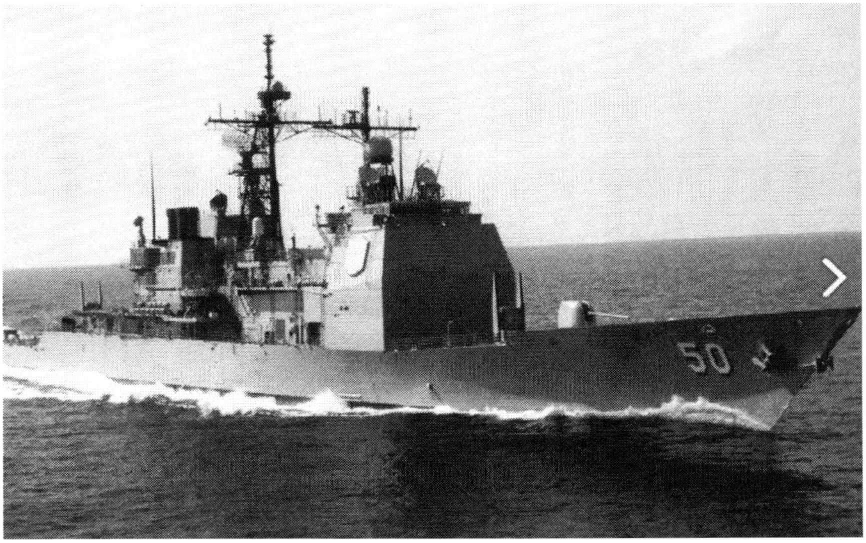

I was very familiar with San Diego because of my time at Chula Vista High School, so I was excited to reunite with some old high school friends. On the other hand, SN Wibberley was excited to return to the East Coast to be closer to his family. If I remember correctly, he was from Pennsylvania. In the end, we ended up with letters of recommendation to attend an "A" school in the near future and hoped that they would be our saving grace. In the following year, I came to find out that SN Wibberley was one of the seventeen sailors killed in the USS Cole (DDG-67) terrorist attack. I was shocked and saddened to see his face in the newspaper.

CHAPTER 2

Get Your Feet Wet First

I reported to USS Valley Forge (CG-50) on October 31, 1999. I had just turned eighteen the month before, and I will never forget the first time I walked on the pier wearing my dress blues while carrying two seabags and a duffel bag. There was a stench in the air near Pier 18: a combination of sewage and a garbage dumpster. The unpleasant smell, combined with vapors randomly shooting out into the air, somewhat reminded me of Gotham City. The most comforting thing about that day was knowing that my buddy from boot camp and seaman apprenticeship training, SN Adrian Arriola, had received the same orders as me.

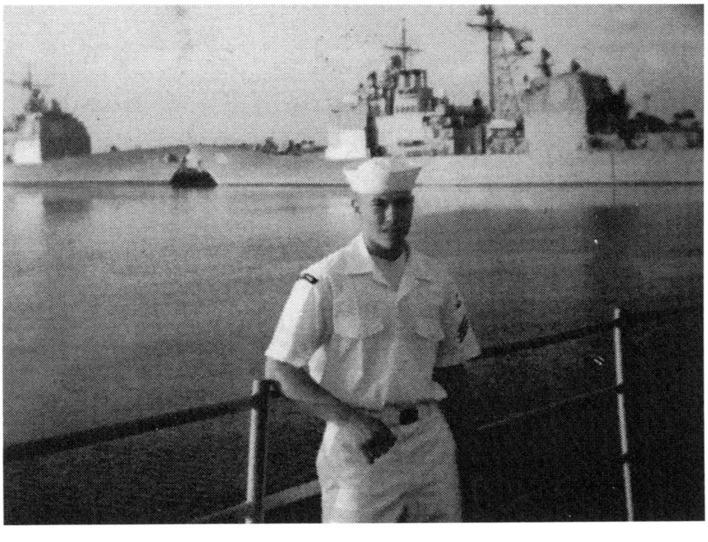

I presented myself at the quarterdeck, just as we were trained to do, and saluted the American flag first and then the Officer of the Deck. The Officer of the Deck reviewed my orders and then had the messenger of the watch escort me to my new living space in aft ops—a compartment I'd share with forty to fifty other sailors. There were only two toilets, two showers, and two sinks, and my bunk felt like a coffin. It was a Friday evening, so the compartment was empty. I was granted liberty for the rest of the weekend but was instructed to return no later than 2200 on Sunday since the ship would be underway come Monday morning. I had reported just in time for the beginning of scheduled underway exercises in preparation for a deployment to South America in March 2000. Being underway with the Navy is not a Disney cruise, as members of other military branches might think; it is a thrilling experience that involves nonstop warfare operations.

On Monday morning, I was delighted to see that the galley had unlimited boxes of cereal to choose from. Cereal was my favorite thing growing up. I would have it for breakfast, lunch, and

even dinner. My parents often joked that if I ever got stabbed, I would most likely leak whole milk instead of blood. After my first breakfast on the ship, I reported to the personnel office. I handed in my military orders and, most importantly, made sure they received a copy of my letter of recommendation for "A" school. The sailor laughed at me and said that the letter of recommendation meant nothing in that environment. He even showed it to one of his peers so he could have a nice laugh, too. I knew at that very moment that I was screwed. I would have to serve my two years alongside other undesignated deck seamen before receiving any healthcare-related training.

Or would I? I was a very persistent kid—maybe more like a pain in the ass—but that usually got me to the places where I wanted to be. In general, I consistently achieved my goals not through smarts but through hard work and perseverance. I knew there had to be a viable way to get closer to becoming an HM. If you want something, then you must do something about it. I knew that spending the next two years sweeping, swapping, chipping, and painting bulkheads was not an option for me.

A few days later, I decided to visit the medical department and introduce myself to the chief petty officer in charge, so I found a door with a red cross on it and knocked. I was convinced that I'd make a good impression, but all of that went down the drain when I was greeted by a stern senior chief petty officer named Peter Espitia. He opened the door and immediately asked, "What can I do for you?"

Of all the many different and intelligent ways I could have articulated my intention, I blurted out, "How can I work here? [with my Laredo accent]."

After establishing where I currently worked and that I'd only been there since the week before, he informed me that I needed to get my feet wet first before switching jobs. He told me to return in six months to see how things were going.

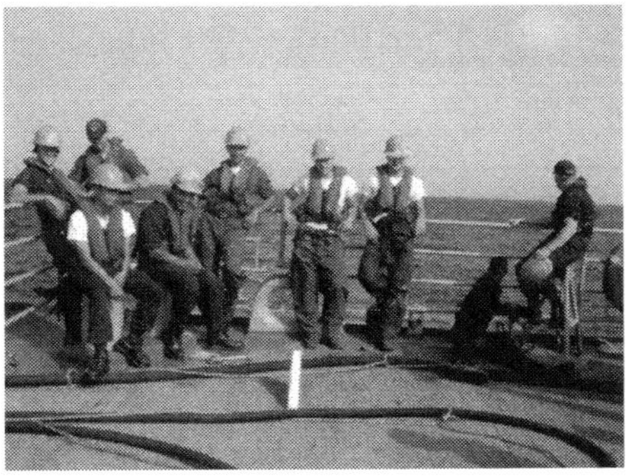

Before I knew it, six months had passed, and we were now headed for a six-month deployment to South America and the Caribbean. We were scheduled to make stops in Mexico, Ecuador, Panama, Aruba, Curaçao, and Florida, then return to San Diego. Working in deck division was more fun than I had imagined. Our job was simple: be where you need to be on time and do what the Boatswain's Mates ask you to do. If they ask you to sweep, you sweep. If they ask you to paint, you paint. If they ask you to do preventive maintenance, you do it. If they ask you to jump off the ship—just kidding—I'm just checking to see if you're keeping up with the deck seaman life. But the highlight of working in the deck division was obtaining my helmsman qualification. Who would have thought that those big ships were all being steered by a bunch of sailors in their late teens and early twenties?

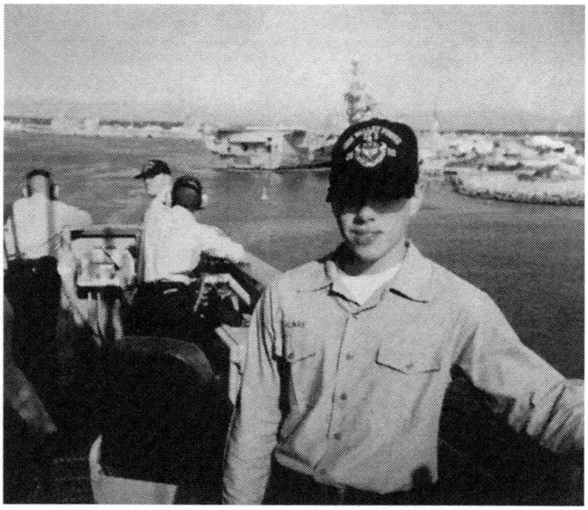

At this point, I felt I had gotten my feet wet and was better prepared to knock on the door with the red cross again. For a second time, HMCS Espitia greeted me at the door. Part of me wanted to say, "Remember me?" Instead, I reminded him that he'd asked me to return after six months and then asked if I could work for him now. He said there was no way my leadership would let me go in the middle of a deployment and that I would have to come back later. I was starting to get the feeling that my notions of training in the medical department were a bit unrealistic and that only a miracle would make it happen for me.

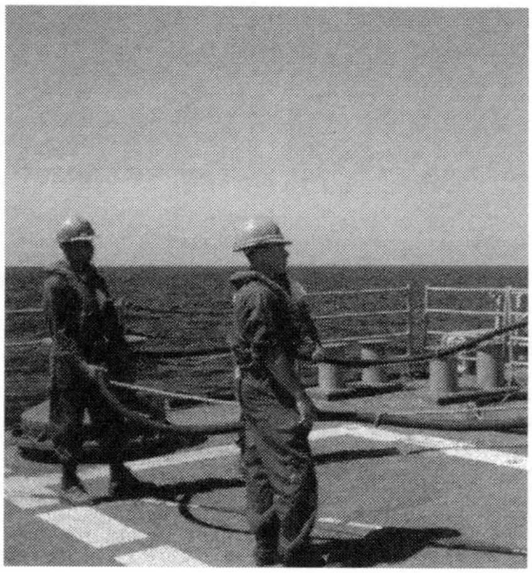

Several weeks after returning from the deployment, I found myself working topside, chipping paint on the starboard (right) side of the ship. I felt a few taps on my right shoulder, and when I turned around, it was HMCS Espitia. He asked if I was still interested in medical work, and I immediately removed my earplugs to make sure I had heard him correctly. He clarified that I needed to speak with my supervisor first, but he could use some help now. Both of his hospital corpsmen had suffered unrelated medical emergencies; Hospital Corpsman 2nd Class Corey Hanson would require an extended convalescent leave, and Hospital Corpsman 3rd Class Joey Lingard had broken an arm and had to wear a cast. He was still planning to work in the medical department but would be significantly limited in what he could do. My department leadership approved the transfer from the deck division to medical.

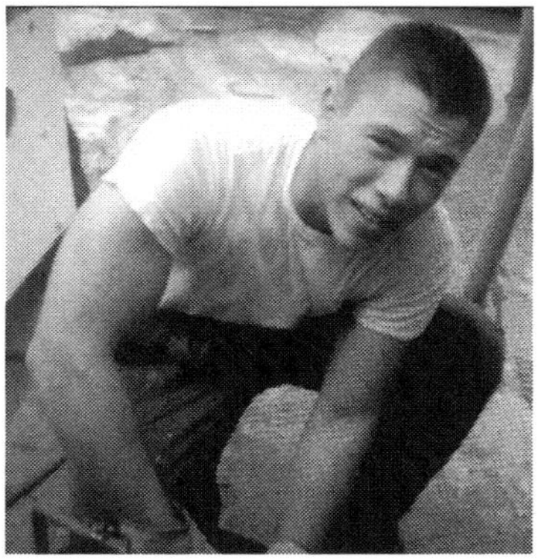

Upon receiving approval to initiate the transfer, HMCS Espitia prioritized getting me trained. I was not a hospital corpsman, but I needed to function as one. In a short period of time, he was able to get me basic life support certified. He taught me how to conduct basic physical assessments, administer intramuscular injections, sterilize surgical instruments with an autoclave, and document subjective, objective, assessment, and plan (SOAP) notes.

The skill that impacted me the most, though, was intravenous (IV) insertion. I just could not understand how it was possible to insert a needle into someone's arm and into a vein to thread a catheter. I found it pretty amusing, actually. He reviewed the procedure several times, but we didn't have any simulation training models with which to practice. Considering HM3 Lingard had only broken one arm, he figured we could use his other arm for IV practice. I went ahead and collected all of my supplies: a tourniquet, an 18-gauge catheter, a 10 cc normal saline (NS) flush, IV tubing, a liter of 0.9% NS, alcohol preps, gauze, and an occlusive site dressing. I spiked the bag of normal saline only to discover that I had forgotten to clamp my tubing first. NS spilled on the floor, and HMCS Espitia expressed in frustration, "Ok, now we have to start all over again because you freakin' got bubbles in the tubing. You have to clamp the tubing first. Come on, we reviewed this."

I got it right the second time.

Next, it was time to magically get this external device into HM3 Lingard's vein. I knew I was going to fail before I even attempted it. The idea of cannulating a vein seemed so unreal to me at the time, but I went for it! And this is more or less how my first stick was narrated: "Hey, that's not how I taught you to put on the tourniquet. Go ahead and stick… stick. Reposition to the right a little bit. That's too much; go a little more to the left. Advance and look for blood return in the chamber. Alright, that's enough. Loosen up your tourniquet and remove the catheter."

Overall, my first IV attempt went exactly how I thought it would. It was unsuccessful in many ways, but the root cause of my lack of confidence was that I hadn't gone through the motions of preparing and inserting the catheter sufficiently before sticking a real human. The reality was that we didn't have the right training tools to do this. It was a ship, not a training center. The best that HMCS Espitia could do was review the steps with me and somewhat simulate how the procedure should play out, then have me attempt the procedure on a human being. That's as real as it gets.

One thing I learned to admire in the Navy was the nonstop training that took place. I don't recall it ever being called simulated training, but that's exactly what it was. A perfect example of this would be the periodic general quarters drills that were conducted with the crew. General quarters is a ship-wide call for all crew members to get in position for battle. It is also known as manning one's battle station. We simulated attacks on our ship so frequently that I knew exactly where to go, what to do, and how quickly I would need to react without a second thought. My training experience aboard USS Valley Forge set the standard for what deliberate practice should look like, regardless of one's profession.

This exposure to the medical field changed my life forever. I was determined to pursue my goal of becoming a medical professional, so with the assistance of the ship's career counselor, Navy Counselor (NC) 1st Class Mark McCoy, I decided to take advantage of a commissioning program called Naval

Reserve Officers Training Corps (NROTC). TM2 Garza, my Navy recruiter, introduced me to this program before I shipped out to boot camp, so I knew it existed. The application asked for simple information like one's demographics, military service, schools attended, academic records, extracurricular activities, and four candidate statements. It was a pencil-filled application, so it felt very similar to taking a test in high school again. I was only a year into my first sea tour and would have nowhere else to go for another year, so I figured I might as well submit an officer package.

As much as I had learned and had fun as a deck seaman, I knew it was time to move on. We were scheduled to enter the shipyard at NASCO in San Diego in the spring of 2001. I knew that both HM3 Lingard and HM2 Corey would soon return to full status and that I would eventually get thrown back into the deck division during the shipyard maintenance period. Aside from going underway, this period is one of the toughest for anyone working as a Boatswain's Mate or deck seaman; that's their bread and butter. So, I did the unimaginable.

The dry-side base on 32nd Street would be holding wrestling tryouts. The top two winners in each weight class would receive temporary assignment orders to train and compete with the South Pacific (SOPAC) Navy Team, a stepping stone to selection for All-Navy Wrestling. I wrestled for Chula Vista High School and lost most of my matches, so what did I have to lose, right? Similar to Diego Maradona's legendary goal against England in the 1986 FIFA World Cup quarterfinals, the "Hand of God" must have been with me on the wrestling mat that day. I won a spot to represent the SOPAC team in 2001.

With the support of my leadership, I was allowed to transfer to the wrestling team on Temporary Assigned Duty (TAD) orders. For the next few months, my job was to train nine hours a day, five days a week, and compete at local and regional tournaments on Saturdays. Maintaining good nutrition was very difficult for me. At nineteen years old, I struggled to make weight at 138 pounds. My usual meals were an apple for breakfast, soup and salad for lunch, a midday snack that was usually a power bar, and an orange for dinner. I always felt weak.

Every evening after wrestling practice, it became my routine to walk up to one of the base pay phones and dial 1-800-NROTC for a status update on the officer package I had submitted the previous year. My parents, who still lived in Laredo, would joke that if selection came down to how many calls an applicant made, then I would certainly take the lead. I called at least once a day for several months. The combination of feeling physically weak and mentally disillusioned due to a lack of news was tough. Then, one day after wrestling practice in the spring of 2001, I dialed as I usually did. Only this time, the recording said, "Congratulations. You have been selected for the 2001 NROTC scholarship." I hung up and froze for a good minute. Was I dreaming? I called again just to make sure, and I had indeed been selected and assigned to the University of California, Los Angeles (UCLA). Finally—an opportunity to pursue my dream of becoming a physician!

"I am sorry to burst your bubble, man, but this program is not going to work out if you're color-blind," said the medical evaluator during my Department of Defense (DoD) Medical Examination Review Board, which is a required physical exam for the final NROTC selection process. "You need to get in touch with your career counselor ASAP to figure out an alternative."

I wanted to punch myself in the face for not reading the medical eligibility qualifications more carefully. I was so focused on the academic and performance aspects that I neglected the color vision stipulation. Color blindness is something that I naturally adjusted to as a child because I didn't even know I was color-blind until I joined the Navy. I remember telling my mom that my teachers at school deducted points from all of my coloring assignments. Once, I asked her for help on a homework assignment involving colors, and she responded, "*No te hagas el menso*!" This translates to, "Don't play stupid!"

My only option at this point was to take the medical evaluator's advice and seek out NC1 McCoy for potential alternatives. NC1 McCoy was a serious man but very helpful and experienced. He took good care of his sailors. When I met with him, he told me I had two options: the Marine Corps or the Navy Nurse Corps (NC). As an ignorant nineteen-year-old, I said, "Let's go with the Marine Corps because nursing is for women." The Marine Corps ended up rejecting me because my personal statement didn't reflect the right values, meaning I wasn't Marine Corps material. So, I bit the bullet and applied for the NC. I wouldn't get the opportunity to join the medical field as a physician, but at least I would be in a related field. The change of program and resubmission of an NC application was accepted, along with a change in school to the University of Texas at Austin. I also received orders to attend HM "A" School in Great Lakes that same week. I recall NC1 McCoy calling me into his office and asking whether I wanted to attend nursing school at UT Austin or HM "A" School in Great Lakes. Without hesitation, I went with Austin to be closer to home.

Since I would soon transfer duty stations, the wrestling team decided it was best that I return to USS Valley Forge to complete my administrative separation. Under the NROTC program, I would need to be discharged from active duty and participate as a civilian. This required a complete separation package, including medical physicals. I returned to USS Valley Forge in May with the news of my officer program selection. I thought it'd be a good idea to request to return to the medical department for some on-the-job training. By this time, most of my original deck division leadership had transferred out to other duty stations, including HMCS Espitia. My request to work in the medical department for the last three months of my time on the ship was denied. Deck division was undermanned and overworked, so I returned to seamanship operations. But this time, I found peace knowing that a new chapter was in sight.

I spent the morning of my last day aboard USS Valley Forge obtaining last-minute approval signatures and saying farewell to shipmates I had learned to call brothers over the last two years. I still keep in touch with guys like Adrian Arriola, Chris Terry, Sam Gutierrez, and Jimmy Diaz to this day.

Lastly, I met with my fellow "deck monkeys," as they called us in the fleet, for a final goodbye. Prior to my departure, my Boatswain's Mate supervisor called us all into the port side smoke break for a quick gathering. As the name implies, it was called the smoke break because that's where sailors were allowed to smoke while the ship was moored to the pier. It was a covered area that could not be seen from an external view. As soon as I entered, I received the good 'ole deck seaman farewell, which translated to kicks and punches until I hit the deck. It was their way of showing love. They picked me up and then, one by one, gave me hugs and Cali-style handshakes. It wasn't the first beating I'd received in my lifetime, so I took it like a champ.

However, the most remarkable moment I remember about that last day was my departure from the ship. It is a naval custom to announce the arrival and departure of the commanding officer (CO) via the 1 Main Circuit (MC), a system used to issue communications throughout the entire ship. For example, when a CO arrives or departs the ship, four bells are rung, followed by a 1MC announcement, "USS Valley Forge, departing/arriving." That day, the command duty officer requested approval from the CO to announce my departure. Similarly, two bells were rung (instead of four), followed by the 1MC announcement: "Seaman Salinas departing."

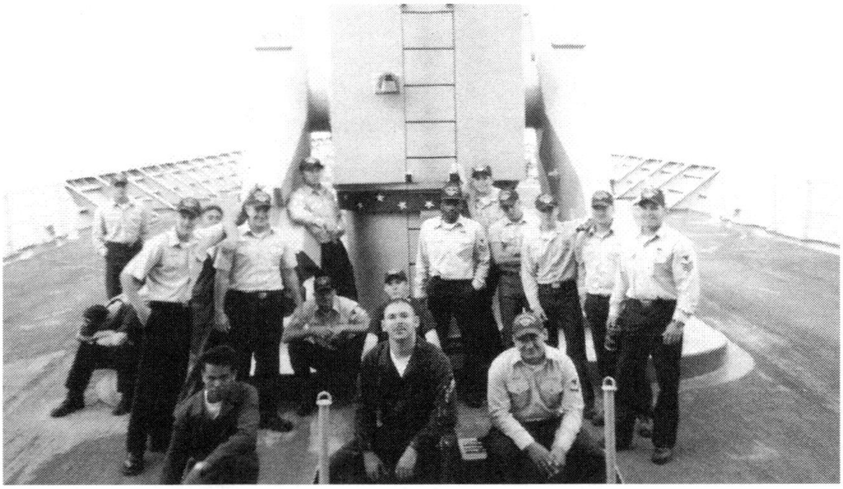

CHAPTER 3

Train Like You Fight

The next four years in Austin were action-packed. My orders were to participate in the Navy/Marine Corps ROTC, maintain at least a 3.0 GPA, and develop as a nursing professional. It sounded straightforward, except that I came to realize that I would have to survive on $250 a month my first year, $300 the second year, $350 my third, and finally, $400 my last year. I was two months shy from hitting my three-year mark as an enlisted member, so I was not entitled to the Montgomery GI Bill that I had paid into throughout my first year on active duty.

I remember purchasing smoothies at Jamba Juice for a straight week with my good friend Marcus Foster, another midshipman in the same predicament. We thought that we would be swimming in cash thanks to the bill. We were wrong. Marcus was much smarter than me, though, and figured out a way to finance a dorm room at the local Castilian. On the other hand, I was living in a house in North Austin with two dudes, Aaron and Paul. It was fun, but it was not sustainable with my limited savings, and I didn't qualify for any other financing. So my parents helped me purchase a 35-foot trailer and station it in a trailer park called Mobile Home Haven. Compared to the navy ship I had recently left behind, a trailer had more room than I needed. My bed had hydraulics that allowed it to be lifted so I could stow clothes and miscellaneous things underneath it, just like I did with my ship's bunk bed.

For food, I used an Exxon gas card that my parents graciously gifted me; frozen sandwiches, bananas, and Snickers bars became my go-to meals. I will never forget the day I overdrew my checking account twice at a gas station when my card was swiped first to purchase a Snickers bar and then again when I decided to add a banana to the tab. If I remember correctly, I was charged $25 per overdraft, which added up to $50 total for a chocolate bar and one banana. The struggle was real.

To offset the financial hardship, I decided to pick up a few jobs. I worked as a mover for a company called ABC Moving, as a nursing assistant on a medical-surgical floor at Brackenridge Hospital (which I recently learned no longer exists), and as a tutor for introductory biology as well as chemistry and nursing courses at a rate of $10 per hour. I also participated in blood donations twice a week for $50—every dollar counted! Nevertheless, my experience as a nursing assistant at Brackenridge was pivotal to my professional growth. Becoming proficient at performing some of the most mundane tasks at the hospital (changing bed sheets, taking vital signs, tracking intake and output, obtaining glucose checks, and assisting with activities related to a patient's daily life) set me up for success as a nursing student.

I always kept in mind two learning concepts that stuck with me from both my shipboard and my wrestling experiences. To be good at anything, one must constantly practice in an environment that resembles the real deal as much as possible. For example, if you want to be a mechanic, you practice on vehicles. If you want to be a chef, you practice in a kitchen. If you want to be a pianist, you practice on a piano. If you want to be a swimmer, you go practice in a pool. If you want to be a medical provider or nurse, however, you can't simply go practice on patients in a clinic or at a hospital. That would be considered unethical, so we turn to simulation. The same thing applies to aviation; you definitely want to practice on a simulator before attempting to fly a passenger airplane because the stakes are too high.

Much of what we know about simulation comes from the aviation industry. The first flight simulator was invented in 1910 and was later in demand for fighter pilots during World War II. Today, simulators are used in many industries, including but not limited to healthcare, military, transportation, law enforcement, sales and retail, construction, and agriculture. I was exposed to a variety of different simulators in the Navy. Whether it was firefighting, damage control, general quarters, mass casualty, or seamanship training, simulation was at the core of it all. When I started nursing school in 2003, simulation was still not as robust as it could have been. Our simulation lab was limited to task trainers that were only adequate for teaching specific skills like inserting Foley catheters, administering intramuscular injections, placing IVs, nasogastric tube insertion, changing dressings, and tracheostomy care. It lacked the comprehensiveness and problem-solving approach that are characteristic of simulation programs in nursing schools today.

Although the aviation industry catapulted simulation methods to the next level in the twentieth century, simulation in healthcare dates back to the Middle Ages when surgical skills were practiced on animal carcasses. More refined task trainers and birthing simulators were later adopted in the 1600s and 1700s, but it wasn't until 1911 that the first nursing manikin, Mrs. Chase, was created. Maternal mortality rates for childbirth were about 1% (that's one death per every hundredth delivery) in the early twentieth century, so it made sense that the world desperately needed a Mrs. Chase. Today, medical simulation works wonders for healthcare quality and safety programs, but we still have plenty of improvements to make, and healthcare is constantly evolving.

In recent years, health professions have embraced immersive VR because of its ability to accelerate learning and seamlessly bridge the gap between theory and practice. Immersive VR is a computer-generated, three-dimensional environment that alters one's perception using simulated environments that make objects and scenes feel real. Notable advantages of

VR include standardization, accessibility, repeatability, and cost-effectiveness.

1. **Standardization:** Consistency during training is crucial. You may have heard the old saying, "There is more than one way to skin a cat." This holds true in some cases, but for the most part, educators ought to be standardizing evidence-based practices and asking, "What does the latest research say about the skills we are attempting to teach, and how do we develop a template to keep the curriculum consistent?" Not only does it alleviate the learner's anxiety by reassuring them that there is a standardized plan for them to gain knowledge and perform a skill, but it also helps the educator by giving structure to their instruction. Have you ever encountered different clinical competency checklists for the same skill at the same facility? I know that I have. Inconsistencies in practice alter clinical outcomes. To produce the same high-quality healthcare professionals, we must advocate for standardization.

2. **Accessibility:** There were countless times during my nursing training during which I felt I could have benefited from additional hands-on training to master a particular skill. I am the kind of person who loses sleep when I feel unprepared. Whether it is competing in sports, giving a presentation, participating in a meeting, or even hosting a house party, unpreparedness leads to anxiety for me. Nursing school simulation labs do not typically have walk-in hours that allow students to hone in on their skills whenever it's most convenient. Simulation time is normally scheduled and coordinated through a simulationist, limiting the number of times a student can practice. Is the expectation that students will eventually get comfortable with knowledge, skills, and attitudes (KSAs) once they get out in the real world? I think we can do better than that.

3. **Repeatability:** Learning experts say it takes the average human being about seven times to transfer content in our brains from short- to long-term memory. For me, sometimes it feels closer to one hundred! But, it is through repetition that new synaptic terminals in our neurons are created. Protein synthesis is accelerated through repetitiveness, leading to sustained memory and improved performance. One of my favorite learning theories, mastery learning, encourages as much repetition as is necessary to successfully meet all milestones or steps of a particular skill sequentially. VR is an excellent environment in which to apply mastery learning principles.

4. **Cost-effectiveness:** Costs associated with starting and maintaining a simulation center are extremely high, ranging from $200,000 to $1.6 million and at least $15,000 for annual maintenance. Considering the financial constraints that haunt academic institutions and hospitals today, full-scale simulation centers are not sustainable solutions for everyone. I am not implying that VR modalities should replace high-fidelity simulation centers; instead, VR should be explored as a supplemental modality to augment traditional healthcare education and training methods. Start-up and maintenance costs for VR education and training programs range between $10,500 and $60,000, depending on the number of headsets, scenarios, and implementation support needed. With that in mind, if I tell you that there is no significant difference in learning outcomes between high-fidelity simulators and VR methods, which would you purchase for your organization?

One thing I really came to appreciate about my nursing program was that it started us all off with learning the most fundamental skill in healthcare—communication. Communication in Healthcare Settings was a prerequisite course that introduced nursing students to empathy, conflict resolution, principles of distance and space, listening, confidentiality, consent, cultural awareness, and more. However, there was little to no opportunity to enhance this skill in a simulated clinical environment prior to the start of actual clinical training. It was mainly didactic. If you were to ask nursing students what the biggest challenges of the clinical setting are, you would receive a variety of different responses: time management, medication administration, procedural skills, and documentation. The hardest part for me was getting comfortable knocking on a patient's door and introducing myself. The thought of walking into someone else's personal space made me feel as if I were intruding on my commanding officer in his stateroom. When I worked in the medical department on the ship, patients came to us; now, I had to go to them.

One nursing home patient helped me break this barrier in 2003. His name was Norman Lafair. He was a WWII pilot veteran who was full of vivid stories that made me feel like I was right there in the thick of it with him. He made me realize that patients were, in fact, real people and that we were there to help them get better, not to be judged by them. During my last visit with Norman, he asked me to help him put his socks on. I knew that we were supposed to wear non-sterile gloves for these types of things, but I decided to skip the gloves and put the socks on with bare hands. I figured that if Jesus Christ could wash crud off people's feet, then I should be able to put clean socks on Norman. He looked at me and said, "Son, you're going to be a great nurse someday."

Dr. Hartzell, my first clinical instructor, transformed how I approached my nursing interventions. I had always been ambitious in school, and it really bothered me that I was only getting in the high 80s on my nursing care plan assignments. After receiving these subpar grades on two consecutive assignments, I scheduled time to meet with her to figure out what I was doing wrong—or, rather, what I could do better. She pointed out that the quality of my work was excellent, but I was missing some key elements in the rationales section. She challenged me to ask why after every intervention. Why is the patient admitted? Why is the patient on antibiotics? Why are we performing neurological checks every hour? Why is the patient on anticoagulants? This was fundamental to developing critical thinking, she'd said. I associated nursing clinical rotations with attending church once per week. On Sunday, you are burning with the Holy Spirit, but by Friday, the only burn you feel is tequila running down your throat. In clinical training, you felt like a real nurse on Monday, but by Sunday, you felt like quitting school. Clinical training must be consistent and easily accessible for students to maintain high confidence levels and improve their critical thinking skills. From that day forward, the word "why" was at the forefront of all my interventions.

I was also learning how to become a naval officer during this time. I had to modify the way I spoke and the way I dressed. After hanging out with deck seamen in Southern California for a couple of years, I must admit that I had picked up some bad habits. There would be no more "wassup, foo" in my vocabulary and no more baggy pants in my wardrobe (or under my trailer's hydraulic bed). Following ROTC rules was a must. Part of Captain (CAPT) Gene Garrett's (the Navy ROTC commanding officer) welcome talk when I first met him in person was to warn me that if I didn't meet the program's standards, I would return to the fleet as an undesignated deck seaman. There was no possible way I would let that happen, so I committed myself to playing the ROTC game and quickly became accustomed to getting yelled at by midshipmen who had no fleet experience, physical training early in the morning, wearing my uniform around campus, and completing mandatory naval college courses. It was a breeze compared to what I had already experienced in the fleet.

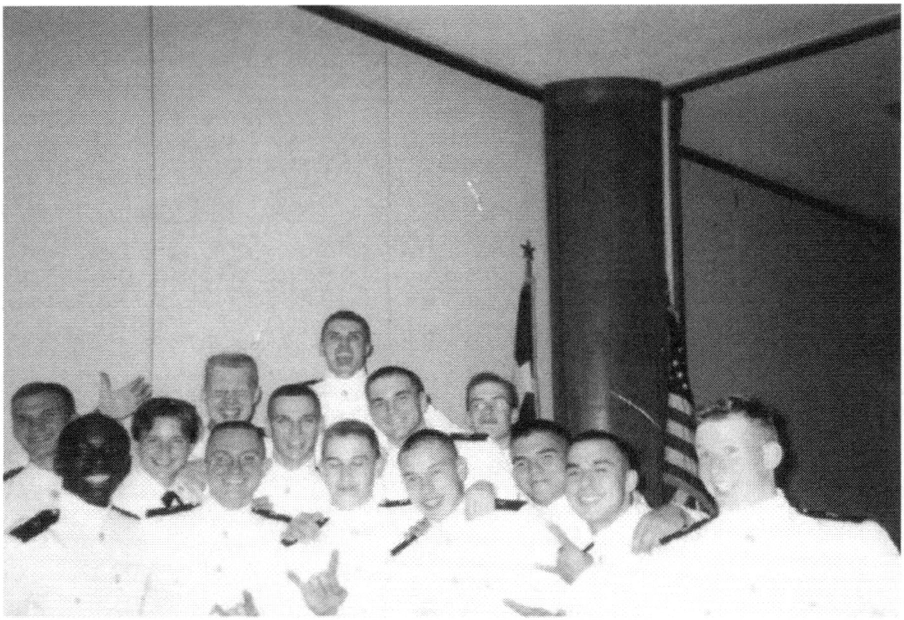

The most vital thing I learned in ROTC was how to shift gears from thinking about what I needed to do for myself to what I needed to do for my sailors. That is what selfless devotion to duty is all about. If you ever read a naval award citation, you will find those exact words in the last paragraph: selfless devotion to duty. Just like the book *Leaders Eat Last* by Simon Sinek states, you must put the interests of your people before your own. That ideal has even carried over into my family life; my wife, my daughters, and even my dog have everything they need, whereas half of my underwear and socks have holes in them.

Over the next few years at UT Austin, I slowly transitioned into becoming a junior naval officer. I maintained a 3.8 cumulative GPA, became vice president of the Hispanic Nursing Association, joined the judo team (my wrestling experience translated very well there), and volunteered at countless community events. The thought of failing and getting sent back to the fleet was motivation enough for me. Like a boxer who would rather not leave the fight's outcome up to the judges, I didn't want my ROTC leadership to doubt my abilities. I don't recall ever hearing about imposter syndrome back then, but that is exactly what I felt. Imposter syndrome is a phenomenon that was first described in 1978 by Suzanne Imes, PhD, and Pauline Rose Clance, PhD, while researching successful women and other marginalized groups. It can be broken down into five different types: the perfectionist, the superhero, the natural genius, the expert, and the soloist. On paper, I was excelling, but internally, I questioned whether I fit in with the rest of my peers. I think a lot of these feelings stemmed from the drastic change of environment; I'd gone from deck seaman to midshipman, with no stages in between.

In addition to my nursing studies, the NROTC-NC option program required the completion of two four-week summer midshipman training evolutions away from home: shipboard officer training (also known as the first summer midshipman cruise, to be completed between freshman and sophomore years) and a nursing internship (to be completed between junior and senior years).

During shipboard training in 2002, two NC-option colleagues and good friends—Marcus Foster and Carmon Russell—were assigned along with me to the amphibious ship USS Tarawa (LHA-1) in San Diego, which ironically happened to be moored right across from USS Valley Forge at Pier 18. What a surreal feeling it was to walk past USS Valley Forge in my officer's summer white uniform. I was back on 32nd Street, only this time, I was there to get a feel for what it was like to serve as a naval officer.

The objective of the first summer midshipman cruise was to give the prospective naval officer a taste of what the ship lifestyle is like, from reveille (a bugle call to wake up in the morning) to taps (a bugle to signal lights out). Midshipmen who were lined up to become surface warfare officers shadowed junior and senior surface warfare officers, and those of us who were slated to become NC officers were assigned to the ship's medical department. Summer midshipman cruises do not always occur at sea and can be quite stale. Luckily, the USS Tarawa was scheduled to depart San Diego and head to Honolulu, Hawaii, near the end of our four-week training evolution.

The one week underway to Hawaii would put us over our training period, so we were given the option to either stay behind in San Diego or join the venture. Marcus, Carmon, and I decided to remain on board and travel someplace we had never been. In the medical department, we assisted with sick calls by performing basic tasks like prepping exam rooms, taking vital signs, documentation, and filing medical records. But the highlight of the experience was participating in mass casualty training that involved managing an amputation, sucking a chest wound, treating burns and an abdominal evisceration (guts hanging out of the body), and dressing minor abrasions. It was a step up from what I had previously experienced on USS Valley Forge. Catastrophic global events during that period of time, such as the terrorist attacks on USS Cole in 2000 and 9/11, reshaped how the military trained us. Things got a lot more real and gruesome, and simulation began to play a vital role in preparing us for that.

In the summer of 2004, I was shipped to Naval Hospital Portsmouth in Virginia, a tertiary care facility that hosted 250 beds, to supplement what I had learned in my first year of nursing school. I had never visited Virginia before, so I was excited to explore its history and natural beauty. The only issue was that my orders didn't authorize a car rental. To make matters worse, I was provided quarters at Portsmouth Naval Shipyard. The crime rate in Portsmouth was so high in those days that even walking off the base was off-limits. Instead, I had to commute via shuttle.

Nevertheless, the experience was invaluable. My clinical rotations included critical care, medical-surgical, emergency, and mental health. I was expected to work eight-hour days Monday through Friday in direct patient care, including two hours per week in lectures and clinical conferences. As opposed to nursing school clinicals, which were limited to one eight-hour day per week, the daily repetition of providing nursing care at Naval Hospital Portsmouth made a world of difference. It helped me gain more confidence in my skills and prepared me to excel in my last year at UT Austin.

On the morning of May 20, 2005, I was commissioned as an ensign in the U.S. Navy. My first salute was rendered by a former USS Valley Forge shipmate, Yeoman 1st Class Julian Enriquez from San Antonio. Julian was there to represent all the "homies" who were not able to attend, so it really meant a lot to me. I considered him a great mentor and friend.

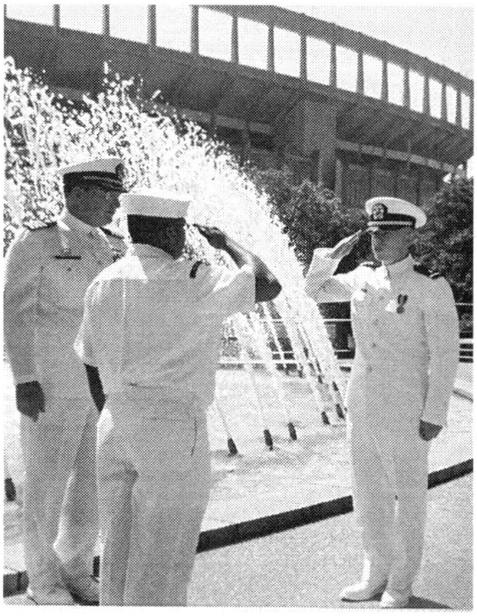

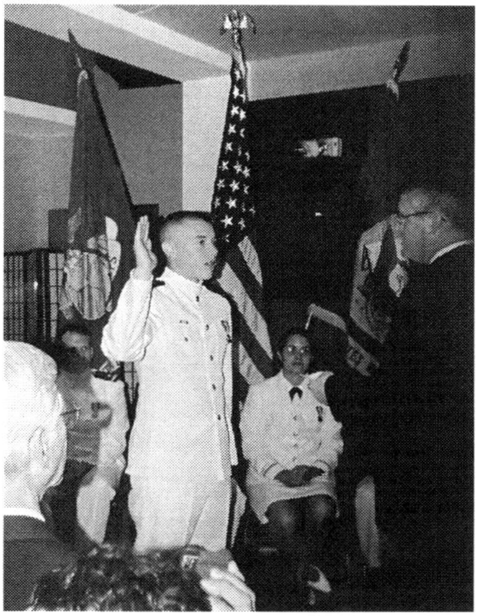

A few minutes after rendering the salute, I rushed myself and my family to the UT School of Nursing graduation ceremony for a special occasion. I didn't have time to change outfits, so I went ahead and threw a cap and gown over my dress white uniform (also known as choker whites) and met with the event organizers backstage. I had been selected to receive the UT Austin School of Nursing Outstanding Bachelor of Science in Nursing Award and I was asked to sit on the stage alongside the faculty. Brigadier General (Ret.) William Bester, the 20th Chief of the Army NC, had recently accepted a faculty position at the UT Austin School of Nursing. He was also backstage to wish me the best in my future endeavors; I still have the military coin he gave me. The most epic moment, however, was when Dean Dolores Sands presented my award and asked me to remove my cap and gown in front of the thousands of attendees at Bass Concert Hall. I removed my cap and gown timidly, in a sort of striptease fashion, to the sound of cheers and applause from the crowd while the NROTC commanding officer, CAPT Donald S. Inbody, presented me with the Distinguished Midshipman Award.

Put It Into Action

Topic/theme	Supporting Evidence	Expected Outcome	Platform
Healthcare Communications	VR enhances realism, helping students better understand patients' perspectives and fostering improved communication skills necessary for collaborative healthcare practice.[1]	Improved confidence with nursing student clinical experiences.	BodySwaps ENGAGE SimX
Undergraduate Nursing Education	VR significantly enhances knowledge acquisition and improves procedural skills in nursing students	Mastery of basic undergraduate nursing skills through repetition (e.g., foley catheter insertion, administering intramuscular	VRPatients SimX ENGAGE TactileVR FacilitateVR

	through repetitive practice.[2,3,4,5,6]	injections, placing IVs, nasogastric tube insertion, changing dressings, and tracheostomy care).	

CHAPTER 4

The Wounded Warriors

My first duty station as a NC officer was the National Naval Medical Center (NNMC) in Bethesda, Maryland, which was renamed Walter Reed National Military Medical Center in 2011.

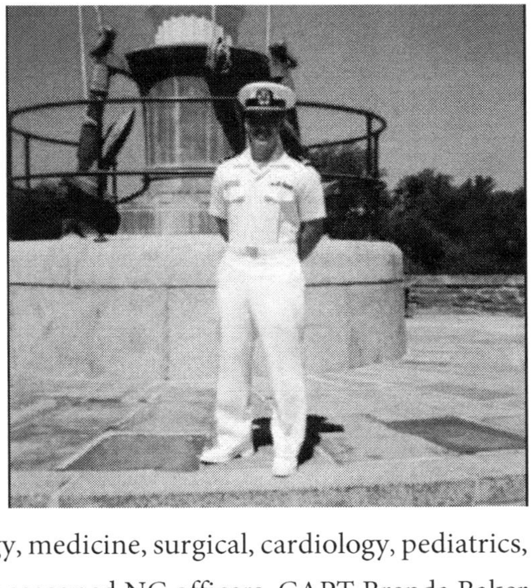

Known as "the President's Hospital," NNMC was the primary hospital for wounded service members from Iraq and Afghanistan to receive medical treatment. Like most hospitals that hire newly graduated registered nurses (RNs), NNMC had a robust ninety-day nurse internship program that exposed novice RNs to various patient care areas, such as oncology, medicine, surgical, cardiology, pediatrics, emergency, and critical care. Two seasoned NC officers, CAPT Brenda Baker and Lieutenant Commander (LCDR) Andrea Petrovanie led the internship program and were instrumental in our professional development. My internship cohort was small (only five RNs), so we benefited from having tailored instruction and flexibility. I didn't have a specific nursing specialty preference prior to my arrival at NNMC, but the internship program changed that. After completing a few rotations, I concluded that oncology was too sad, medicine was too complex, cardiology was too specialized, and pediatrics was just definitely not for me. I mostly preferred to work with adults, so the multiservice surgical ward (5 East) was the perfect fit.

The surgical floor hosted forty-four beds and admitted all wounded warriors who did not meet the criteria for admission to the intensive care unit (ICU). NNMC didn't have a step-down unit, so it was either the ICU or 5 East: nothing in between. That meant that the ward would be fast-paced and challenging. The most common combat-related injuries we treated included amputations, gunshot wounds, shrapnel injuries secondary to improvised explosive devices (IEDs), traumatic brain injuries, and minor burns. RNs on 5 East were required to keep their nursing skills sharp at all times and to become proficient with managing chest tubes, external fixators, patient-controlled analgesia, epidurals, tracheostomies, nasogastric and gastrostomy tubes, bladder irrigation, burn care, blood transfusions, total parenteral nutrition, negative pressure wound therapy, skin grafts, lumbar drains, central lines, and performing vascular access. The majority of wounded warriors required a combination of these skills at any time. I knew that 5 East was where I belonged, so it was my first choice at the end of my internship. My request was granted.

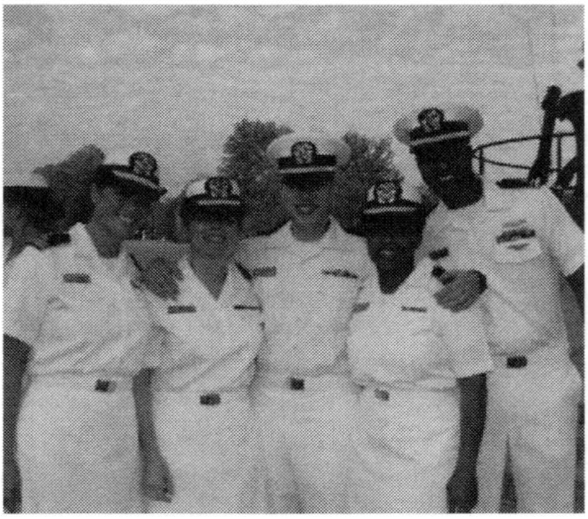

Unlike the internship program, 5 East didn't have a well-structured onboarding program to facilitate the transition. Novice RNs were paired up with other beginners: the blind leading the blind, as some might say. Onboarding was not intentionally set up that way, but the fact was that about 70% of Navy RNs possessed less than two years of clinical experience. The expectation was that we would learn quickly and then return the favor to those who followed us, just like the "see one, do one, teach one" ideology implies. Nevertheless, we never compromised patient safety because we all worked as a cohesive team.

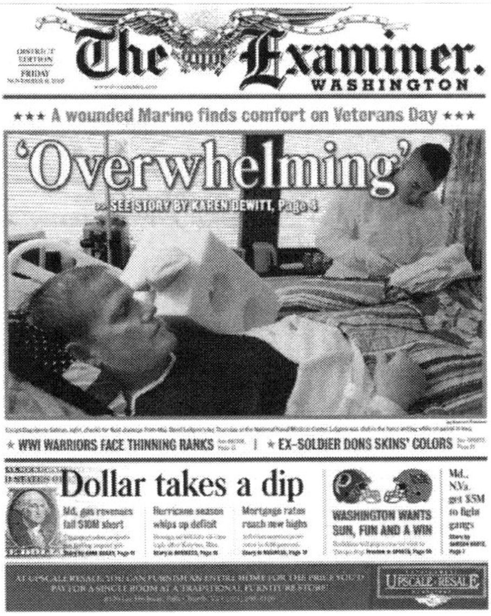
The Examiner.
WASHINGTON
★★★ A wounded Marine finds comfort on Veterans Day ★★★
'Overwhelming'
★ WWI WARRIORS FACE THINNING RANKS | ★ EX-SOLDIER DONS SKINS' COLORS
Dollar takes a dip
Md. gas revenues fall $10M short
Hurricane season whips up deficit
Mortgage rates reach new highs
WASHINGTON WANTS SUN, FUN AND A WIN
UPSCALE RESALE

Within six months, I qualified and assumed duties as charge RN, a role that would normally take a few years for a civilian to take on. Between 2005 and 2007, I witnessed the number of casualties admitted to 5 East rise, which meant that the conflict overseas had intensified.

One of those casualties was Staff Sergeant Jose Pequeño of the New Hampshire National Guard, who suffered a severe brain injury on March 1, 2006, because of an IED blast that left him unable to care for himself.

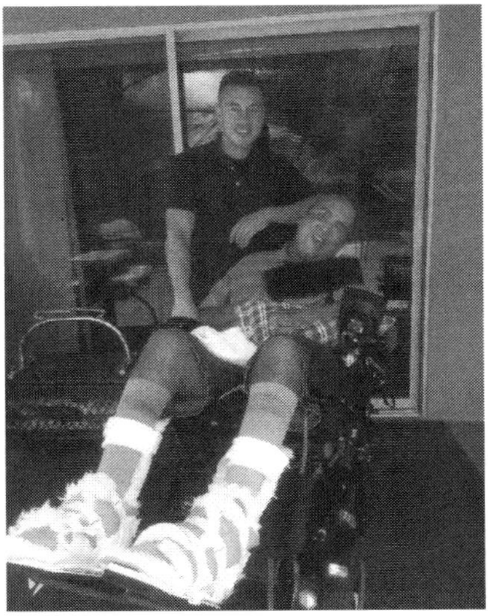

Jose and his mother, Nelida Bagley, became part of the 5 East family during their extensive hospital stay. I had never before experienced the true meaning of motherly love before. Nelida was Jose's biggest champion, and it was up to the 5 East RNs to keep up the fight whenever she wasn't around. If I hadn't learned the meaning of empathy before meeting Jose and Nelida, I definitely learned it then.

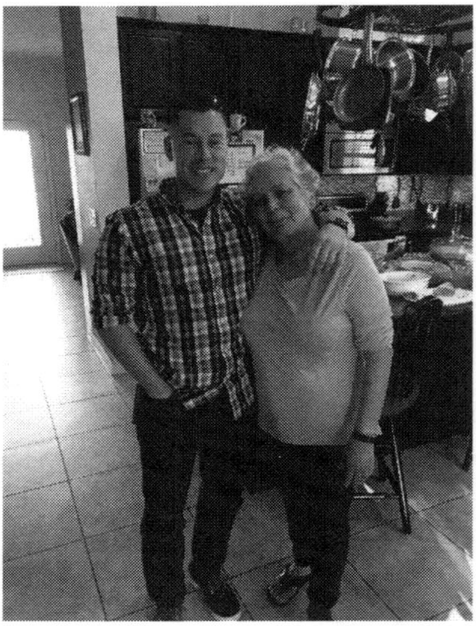

A funny memory that I have is of the day that Nelida asked me to start a new IV in Jose. His veins had progressively gotten worse from the hundreds of IVs he had already had, so it was a special request. By then, I had already become one of the IV experts on the floor, so I was fairly confident in my vascular access skills. I remember Jose's arms being very contracted that day, making it difficult to start an IV the traditional way. So, I decided to insert an IV while upside down to access the only vein I could palpate. It worked, but I made a bloody mess, resulting in Jose's sister, Elizabeth, fainting and falling to the floor. There I was, trying to secure a difficult IV while calling for assistance. In the end, everything was fine, and we were all able to get some good laughs from it.

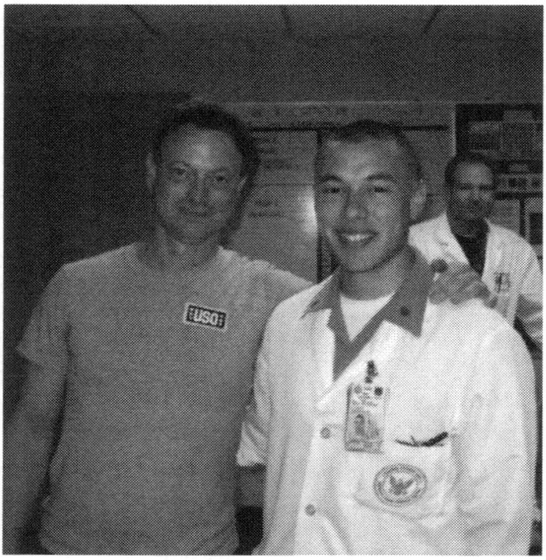

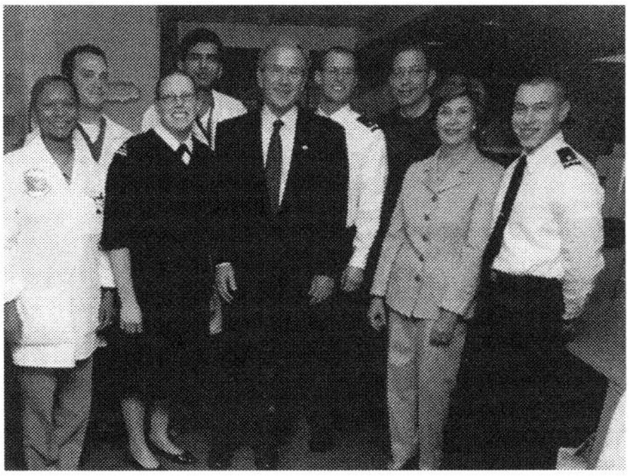

One of the biggest perks of working on 5 East was meeting people that I never imagined I would. The Wounded Warrior Project exemplified the meaning of sacrifice, so it attracted a lot of politicians and celebrities. During my tenure on 5 East, I met President George W. Bush twice, Secretary of Defense Donald Rumsfeld, Secretary of State Condoleezza Rice, Stevie Nicks, Cyndi Lauper, Gary Sinise (Lieutenant Dan), and Benjamin Buford (Bubba) from *Forrest Gump*, the Beach Boys, NFL referees, UFC fighters, and a lot of country singers.

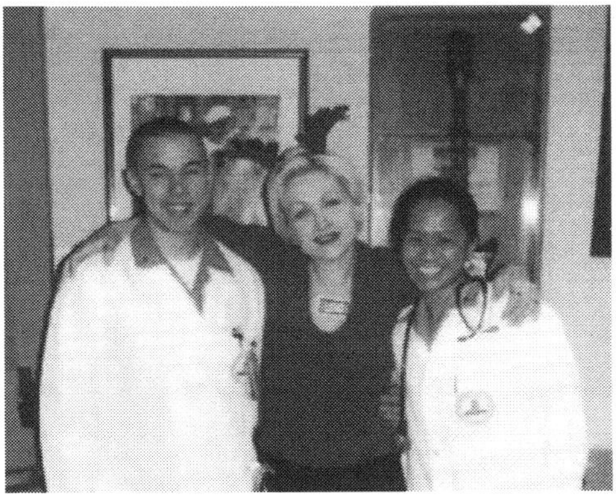

My favorite celebrity of them all was Cyndi Lauper. Not only did she visit each wounded warrior, but she actually sang a song to them. As she was getting ready to leave the floor, I remember jokingly asking, "Hey, what about me? Can I get a song, too?" She turned around and said, "Of course, I can sing a song for you." I couldn't believe it! Lieutenant Junior Grade (LTJG) Aubrey Hall and I were invited to the 5 East family room for a private performance of "All Through the Night." What a great song!

The day-to-night shift rotations every three months, coupled with an average nurse-to-patient ratio of 1:8, were the perfect recipe for staff burnout. It was important for everyone to have an outlet. Some enjoyed traveling, dancing, geocaching, skiing, biking, or hiking, and some even took on the challenge of completing their first full marathon. My good friend Pete Sunden and I decided to sign up for the 2007 Marine Corps Marathon, which was scheduled to take place on October 28, 2007, in Washington, D.C. Pete was also training for Basic Underwater Demolition/SEAL training, so we often worked out together. I will admit that many of those "training" sessions involved drinking pints of beer in Alexandria, Virginia, and then biking back to Bethesda.

The Capital Crescent Trail, which connects Silver Spring, Maryland, to Georgetown in D.C., was near my apartment complex, making it convenient for extended runs and biking. The trail was serene and lined with trees that provided good shade. One late afternoon, as I was on my way back from a run, I ran into an unexpected but familiar face: Brigadier General (Ret.) William Bester. He was also on a run and had apparently accepted a call to serve in a top leadership position at the Uniformed Services University of the Health Sciences (USUHS) in Bethesda. USUHS was right next to NNMC and continues to be the home of the military medical school, the graduate school of nursing, the postgraduate dental college, and allied health sciences even today. Bill, as he liked to be called, suggested we meet over beers in town to catch up. I took him up on the offer a couple of weeks later and met with him at Guapo's Restaurant, located right off Wisconsin Avenue.

The pep talk from someone who had already been there and done that was very much needed. Bill was a genuine leader who enjoyed listening to people. That night, over Budweisers, he told me his personal secret to leadership; one of the things he enjoyed most about his days as Chief of the Army NC was showing up to work early in the morning to shoot the breeze with his staff, including housekeeping personnel. Every single team member played a vital role in the mission, and it was important for him to know how they were all doing. From that day forward, I approached leadership differently. It wasn't about what others could do for me but what I could do for them. His principle paralleled John F. Kennedy's famous line from his 1961 inaugural address: "Ask not what your country can do for you—ask what you can do for your country."

The impact that surgical procedures had on patients amazed me. We would send them to the operating room (OR), and they would magically return all fixed up. Surgery was somewhat mysterious to me because I had never worked in the OR. The perioperative environment was considered too specialized for nursing school and, therefore, was not an option during the internship. I knew nothing about perioperative nursing, but I did come across a few fellow NC officers who spoke highly about the Certified Registered Nurse Anesthetist (CRNA) program. Many of them described this specialty as the pinnacle of nursing because of the highly specialized training it required. CRNAs are advanced practice registered nurses who administer anesthesia for practically all types of surgical procedures. The idea of pursuing a career as a CRNA sounded fascinating, but a hard requirement was to have at least one year of critical care experience under your belt. At that time, there were several different ways to meet the critical care requirement: work in the ICU, emergency room, neonatal intensive care unit (NICU), labor and delivery, or operating room. At NNMC, all of these were viable options except the OR because there was a selection process to attend a perioperative nurse training course in either Camp Pendleton, California, or Jacksonville, Florida. Initially, I decided to transfer from 5 East to the ICU, but the ICU was not accepting transfers at the time of my request.

So, I shifted my attention to the NICU. I was told it was just like the ICU but with neonates. My leadership was very supportive of my professional goals, so they approved the transfer. I remember my first day in the NICU very well. I had never worn scrubs before, so I grabbed cranberry scrubs in what appeared to be my size, but they were small. I presented myself to the NICU's department head with chorizo-tight scrubs. She looked me over from top to bottom and said, "Please go change into bigger scrubs and come back." It didn't take long to figure out that this was nothing like anything I had ever done before. It was a very delicate and serious environment, an about-face from what I had become accustomed to at 5 East; no more VIP visits or fun and games.

The type of empathy I developed working with adults was not the same style of empathy that was needed around devastated parents. It was simply not a good fit for my personality, even though I really enjoyed the critical thinking aspect of working in the NICU. A week before the end of orientation, I cared for a twenty-four-week-old neonate who was not doing very well. His lungs were not mature enough to sustain life without a ventilator, and he was slowly showing more signs of decompensation during my shift. One of my initial interventions was to call respiratory therapy to help clear his endotracheal tube of excess secretions, which quickly turned into a resuscitation effort. We were able to sustain the neonate only long enough for his parents to see him alive one last time. I took some time to process everything and wondered if there was anything I could have done to prevent what happened. I was not ready for this. Later that afternoon, I requested to return to the adult world.

My plan to apply to CRNA training directly from NNMC was not going to work out after all; my time there was running out, and there was no way that I would meet the one-year critical care requirement prior to selecting military orders. Instead, I decided to explore my curiosity regarding the OR by shadowing perioperative RNs. I didn't want to make the same mistake I made when I requested to work in the NICU without ever setting foot in one, so I invested forty off-duty hours in learning about the perioperative environment. Per definition, the term perioperative includes all of the phases of surgery: preoperative, intraoperative, and postoperative. Every surgery I witnessed differed in complexity, but the one thing they all shared in common was teamwork. The constant interplay between the preoperative staff, anesthesia providers, surgeons, surgical techs, perioperative RNs, pharmacists, laboratory and X-ray techs, and postoperative staff made the job very appealing to me. The OR definitely seemed like my kind of place, so I decided to pursue the perioperative specialty.

In early 2008, I received orders to attend perioperative training in Jacksonville, followed by an ultimate duty station transfer to Okinawa, Japan. The perioperative training program was led by LCDR Craig Cunningham, one of the sharpest naval leaders I have ever worked with. There were only two perioperative training programs in the Navy, so the instructors were always selected from a highly qualified pool of candidates. The twelve-week perioperative program consisted of forty hours of didactic education (AORN Guidelines for Perioperative Practice), plus circulating and scrubbing in on a variety of surgical procedures.

I got off to an itchy start during my first week in Jacksonville—literally. There was no lodging available at Naval Air Station Jacksonville, so I ended up booking a room at the Days Inn in Orange Park. Within a couple of days, I ended up with hundreds of bed bug bites on my arms, legs, abdomen, and back. Luckily, our cohort was not scheduled to scrub in on any surgical case until week two of training, which left me just enough time to let the bed bug bites heal.

LCDR Cunningham's teaching method began with the fundamentals and then built from there. In other words, gain the knowledge first before attempting to perform the skill. In terms of surgery, this makes a lot of sense. I can't imagine a surgeon scrubbing in on a case without first knowing the anatomy, physiology, and pathophysiology of the body part(s) they were expected to work on. We were not in the perioperative program to become surgeons, but we needed to think like them. Anticipation was key to becoming a successful perioperative RN, and this mainly boiled down to having whatever the surgeon needed for the procedure available before they even asked for it. Some things, however, can't be anticipated.

For example, the first surgical case I ever circulated was an elective colonoscopy in which the surgeon struggled to maintain insufflation of the colon for visualization. For lack of better words, the air was exiting the butt as quickly as it was going in. The frustrated surgeon paused, scanned the OR, looked at me, and said, "Hey, you. Are you a student?" When I said, "Yes," he replied, "Then come over here and hold this man's butt cheeks together so that I can finish this thing." My job for the next ten or fifteen minutes of my first OR experience was to squeeze a man's butt cheeks together; never would I have anticipated having to do this.

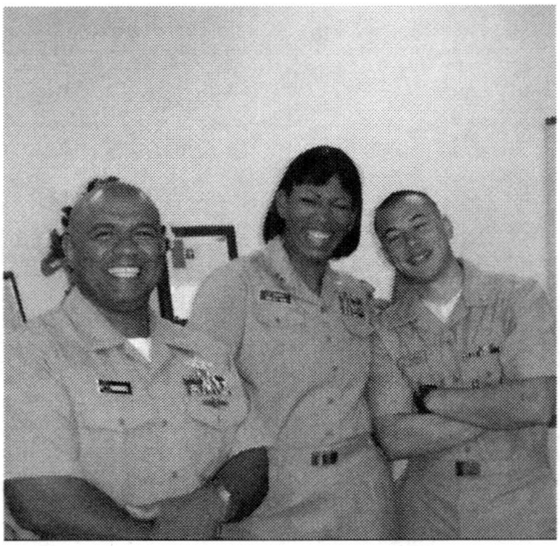

In addition to learning the fundamentals, one of my priorities was to understand the perioperative process. To learn how to effectively anticipate, one must first learn the entire sequence of events that take place in the OR: verifying availability of supplies, equipment, and instrument sets the day before, checking operability of the equipment (including lights, suction, and environmental controls) the morning of procedure, interviewing the patient or legal guardian, opening instrument sets and sterile supplies, performing item counts as needed, transporting and transferring the patient onto the OR bed, securing the patient, assisting with induction of anesthesia, prepping the patient with the appropriate antiseptic solution, helping surgeons gown and glove, performing surgical time-outs, keeping an eye out throughout the procedure, giving a report to the receiving postoperative RN, performing item counts again before closing, transporting to recovery, and performing a safe handoff.

There are often a hundred things going on simultaneously that one must also learn to manage efficiently. But, one of the most challenging tasks was memorizing the dozens of instruments used in surgery, along with their functions. This wasn't because they were inherently difficult to memorize but because instruments were not always accessible for practice. As I mentioned, it takes the average human beïng about seven repetitions to transfer information from short- to long-term memory. Nevertheless, the program was effective and helped us gain the confidence we needed to begin our new journeys as perioperative RNs.

Put It Into Action

Topic/theme	Supporting Evidence	Expected Outcome	Platform
Nursing Skills	VR effectively improves cognitive, psychomotor, and affective performance in novice and experienced RNs. Additionally, VR can serve as an alternative or complementary to traditional didactic delivery methods.[7,8,9,10]	Standardization of initial and ongoing nursing competencies in the clinical setting.	VRPatients SimX 3D Organon BodySwaps Oxford Medical Simulation Tactile VR Lumeto
Perioperative Nursing	Perioperative technical skills, such as laparoscopic navigation and total joint replacement procedures, can be improved through VR.[11,12]	Improve technical skills in surgical techs, operating room nurses, and surgeons.	PeriopSim Metaverse-based platforms
Empathy Development	Immersive VR can accelerate empathy development by	Enhance empathy development in	BodySwaps

	making learners "feel" what it is like to be in someone else's shoes.[13,14]	healthcare professionals.	Metaverse-based platforms
NICU Nursing	VR can improve knowledge, skills, and confidence of NICU healthcare professionals.[15,16,17,18]	Enhance healthcare professionals' confidence by exposing them to essential cognitive and psychomotor skill sets required in the NICU. This is important because NICU clinical rotations are not typical of undergraduate nursing programs.	FacilitateVR SimX

CHAPTER 5

Ganbatte (Give It Your All!)

The flight to Japan felt like an eternity, and I promised myself not to return to the U.S. for the next three years of my tour unless it was absolutely necessary. I must have done about 10,000 calf raises during the flight to keep my blood flowing and to prevent blood clots in my legs. Before the flight, I had heard a story of an airline pilot who flew overseas and developed deep vein thrombosis (DVT) in his lower legs. I didn't want the same type of story circulating about me in the news, so I remained active for eighteen hours straight. Culture shock struck me the moment I landed at Haneda Airport. The staff had the best customer service, and their TSA-equivalent personnel were as respectful as possible. Better yet, the flight attendants bowed before the plane departed for Okinawa and even distributed blankets to each passenger. Google reviews were not a thing back then, but I definitely would have given Nippon Airways five out of five stars.

Okinawa is a breathtaking island renowned for its rich cultural heritage and military history. During World War II, the Battle of Okinawa (which lasted from April to June of 1945) was one of the bloodiest battles in the Pacific Theater and was primarily fought by American troops and the Japanese Imperial Army. It was and continues to be a strategic military post for the U.S. Armed Forces. I was assigned to work at Naval Hospital Okinawa from 2008 to 2011, located on Camp Lester between Kadena Air Force Base and Camp Foster. Since February 28, 1977, Naval Hospital Okinawa has served active duty personnel and their family members, civilian employees, contract personnel, and retirees living on Okinawa. I was pretty anxious about starting a new specialty but excited to hear that five of my good friends from NNMC Bethesda would also be joining me overseas: Pete Sunden (ICU), Danielle Fischer (ICU), Vanessa Franada (multi-service unit), Rob Cuento (multi-service unit), and Pat Parker (OR).

My first day in the OR was hilarious. Pat and I were asked to introduce ourselves at morning muster (our team huddle). This caught me off guard, so I started off by saying, "I am not twenty." I tend to revert to silly humor when I am nervous, but I felt like I needed to get that off my chest because people there seemed to think I was a young enlisted staff member. I hadn't physically changed much since leaving USS Valley Forge.

Someone in the group yelled out, "Well, you're going to look forty by the time you leave this place!"

When it was Pat's turn, he kicked it off by saying, "I am twenty."

He was actually in his early forties and had already experienced Okinawa as a young HM in the 1990s. The OR team had a pretty good laugh, and from that day forward, Pat and I became inseparable at and outside of work.

If one does not already feel dumb before working in the OR, one will definitely experience what it feels like when they first get started. It's because the nature of the environment includes a learning curve so steep that it takes quite a bit of experience to figure out what you are actually doing. I can think of two very embarrassing moments in the OR that made me want to go back to kindergarten.

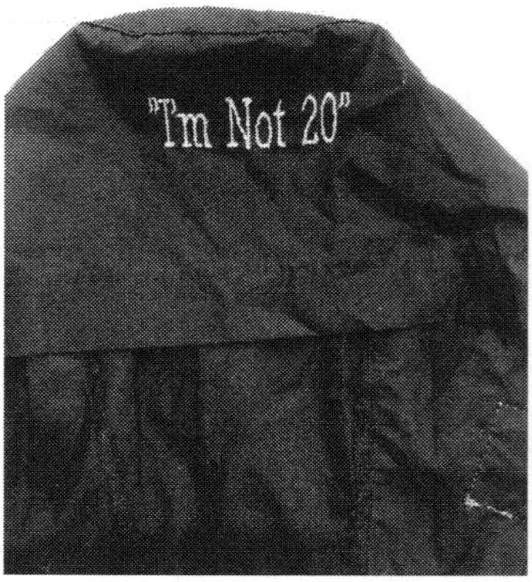

The first occurred during an open inguinal hernia repair. Dr. Adnan Alseidi (now a professor of clinical surgery at the University of California, San

Francisco) was preparing the inguinal site for a PROLENE™ mesh implant when he asked for bacitracin to be added to the mesh. I didn't know what kind of bacitracin he was asking for, and I didn't even bother to ask because I noticed a few boxes of unopened bacitracin ointment in the room and figured that had to be what he wanted. I confirmed with the surgical tech that it was the correct type of bacitracin, and he nodded. A few minutes later, Dr. Alseidi said, "What the heck is this? Bacitracin ointment? Come on, guys!" Thankfully, the mesh never made it to the patient. Dr. Alseidi was asking for a sterile bacitracin solution to dip the mesh into before suturing it in place.

The second dumb moment happened during a laparoscopic appendectomy. In this case, Dr. Travis Polk (now director of the Combat Casualty Care Research Program for the DoD) requested that both of the patient's arms be tucked. This is a standard request because extended arm boards can get in the way of the surgeon standing next to the patient. I was still undergoing orientation in the OR and had just completed a few days of working with the ear, nose, and throat (ENT) team, so I decided to tuck the patient's arms the ENT way: wrapping the patient's upper body (shoulders to fingertips) with a draw sheet. Dr. Polk walked in to assess the patient one last time before scrubbing in and noticed what I'd done. He chuckled and said, "How am I supposed to perform a laparoscopic procedure on a patient who is wrapped in a drawsheet?" I realized then that I had tucked the arms incorrectly for that type of procedure. Even the anesthesiologist provider got a good laugh out of it.

It was not until my twelve-month mark that I had a Private Gomer Pyle "aha" moment, and everything began to make sense. I came to realize that the perioperative process was essentially the same regardless of procedure. All that really changed were the types of equipment, instruments, supplies, and patient positioning techniques required. The cognitive load of a novice perioperative RN was heavier than I had anticipated, so at first, it was challenging to see the big picture. However, daily repetition and exposure to a wide variety of surgical cases made all the difference in the world, which eventually led to proficiency in circulating through the different specialties: general, orthopedic, neurosurgery, obstetrics and gynecology, ENT, oral maxillofacial, ophthalmology, urology, and podiatry surgical cases. I refused to ever feel dumb again, so I made it a habit to dedicate an hour or so at the end of each day to rehearse my flow for the assignments I knew I'd have the next day. Preparation is key in the OR!

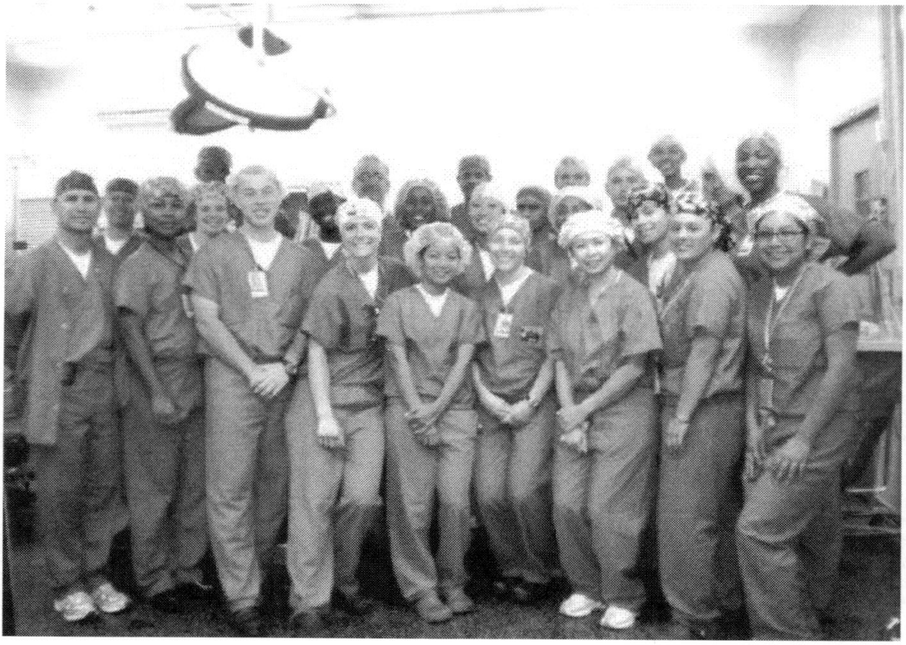

It was not long before the 463 square miles of the island made me feel like I was getting strangled by an anaconda. I felt trapped even though there were tons of different things to do. Like many others, I picked up scuba diving as a hobby. Both Pete Sunden and Dr. Alseidi were avid scuba divers, so I decided to join them on their sea ventures. Shortly after getting my open water diver certification, Dr. Alseidi and some of his local friends invited me on a shore diving trip. The weather conditions were suboptimal for diving, but I trusted that group of guys and joined them off the northwest coast of Okinawa, near Ie Island. Water activities have always had a tendency to make me hungry, so I ate a couple of rice cake snacks on the drive there—a decision I would later regret.

A shore dive meant that we would all have to walk into deeper water before putting on our fins. From a distance, we could see the choppy water crashing against the reef, so we had a rough idea of where the shallow spots ended and the water got deeper. We started walking toward the end of the reef as a group while I made small talk with one of Dr. Alseidi's Japanese friends. I practiced my Nihongo anytime I found the opportunity; I only knew a few phrases, but Japanese people always seemed to appreciate the attempt. Phrases like, *ohayou gozaimasu* (good morning), *konnichiwa* (hello), *toire wa doko desu ka?* (where's the bathroom?), and *biiru futatsu kudasai* (two beers, please) were my "go-to's" anywhere I went. I even knew the word for danger: *abunai*. I used this word to describe the choppy water ahead of us to my new friend. He chuckled and said, "*Dago-san, ganbatte!*" I interpreted that as, "Hey, stop worrying, you can do it!"

And then it happened. We got slammed by a large wave that separated us all, followed by a riptide effect that sucked us all into the deeper water. I had no idea where my fins went, and I struggled to keep my head above water. The weights on my swimsuit were pulling me down just as effectively as my body mass, and I was too inexperienced to consider dropping them to avoid a fight with gravity. I wanted to get out of there, but the current was too strong. I will never forget the memory of seeing the beach and palm trees about 200 meters away and thinking, *Man, I can't believe I'll end up dying in Okinawa.* All I had left was waving my right arm from side to side, hoping someone would see me and help. Out of nowhere, Dr. Alseidi came to the rescue. He pumped my buoyancy control device (BCD) with more air to help me stay afloat; another rookie mistake was not inflating it before the dive. Everyone else had managed just fine, but I had gone into panic mode, thinking this was the end. Moments later, the rice cake snacks that I had enjoyed on my way to Ie were donated to the sea creatures. Never again did I scuba dive in Okinawa.

On December 1, 2009, President Obama announced the deployment of an additional 30,000 troops to Afghanistan to neutralize the proliferation of terrorists in the Middle East. This also meant sending more medical support, but I never considered the possibility of getting deployed from an overseas assignment. A big misconception that was circulating back then was that living overseas was considered being forward-deployed, meaning that one would be exempt from any other types of deployments. But then I received orders to deploy to Afghanistan. On paper, I probably would not have been anyone's first choice due to inexperience (I only had a little bit more than a year of OR experience by that point), but I was the only eligible service member in my department, as two others had been deemed ineligible due to medical conditions.

A lot of questions and thoughts ran through my head. *What type of job will I be doing? Who will I be deploying with? Where in Afghanistan will I be? Will I get a chance to visit my family before leaving? How ironic would it be if I ended up getting injured and admitted as a patient to 5 East at NNMC Bethesda?* I figured it would be more honorable to die for my country in Afghanistan than to drown while scuba diving in Okinawa. My good friend Pete Sunden had also been selected to deploy, and I often wondered if our paths would ever cross in Afghanistan.

In March of 2010, I found myself en route to Tiger Land in Fort Polk, Louisiana, for medical combat advisor training. I had no idea what that meant, but I knew it was something unconventional. In the 1960s, Tiger Land was known by the U.S. Army as "the birthplace of combat infantrymen for Vietnam." It was where soldiers trained in infantry tactics in preparation for the war. In the 2000s, Fort Polk was one of the military sites where medical combat advisors were trained to support Operation Enduring Freedom. In the navy, this meant learning how to speak, dress, and act like a soldier, which entailed completing training in weapons (M2, M240, M249, MK19, M4, and M9), combat patrol under live fire, mine-resistant ambush-protected vehicle (MRAP) driving, land navigation, and combat lifesaving. Additionally, the training involved learning Dari, the official language of Afghanistan, and role-playing with Afghan actors. The quality of training was impressive; it was the best military training I ever received.

The amount of simulation used was the one thing that made all of these training sessions special and different. Simulation was practically used in every training evolution: combat, trauma, and village and leadership engagements. I can't imagine how many millions of dollars were invested at Fort Polk to simulate the real deal. It was not a pretty place at all, but the training made up for the lackluster area. The only good thing about Fort Polk, geographically speaking, was its proximity to my family in Houston. After I completed training, I had the opportunity to travel to Houston over a weekend to bid farewell to my family. On my last night, my Houston cousins decided to take me and a couple of Navy friends (Matt "M12" Marcinkiewicz and Jonathan Fowler) out for some drinks in the downtown area.

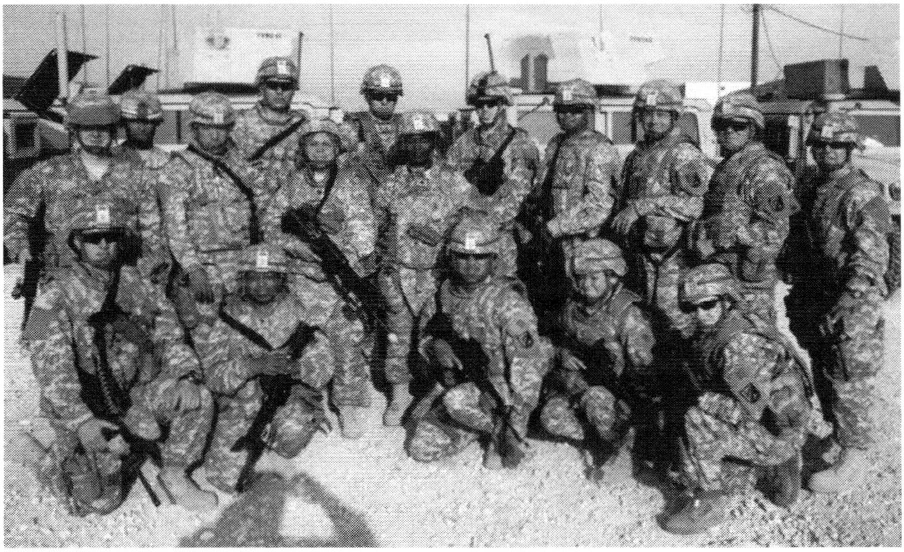

We were having a great time and minding our own business until a fight broke out between two women. It started at the table right next to ours, so we all stood up to get out of the way. We still don't know exactly how it happened, but a woman's purse was thrown high in the air during the fight and coincidentally landed in my cousin Omar's arms. Of course, this would happen to Omar. One of the women immediately falsely accused my cousin of stealing her purse, and we got booted out of the venue by security. It was a pretty funny way to end the night, and it is a story that we still reminisce about every time we see each other.

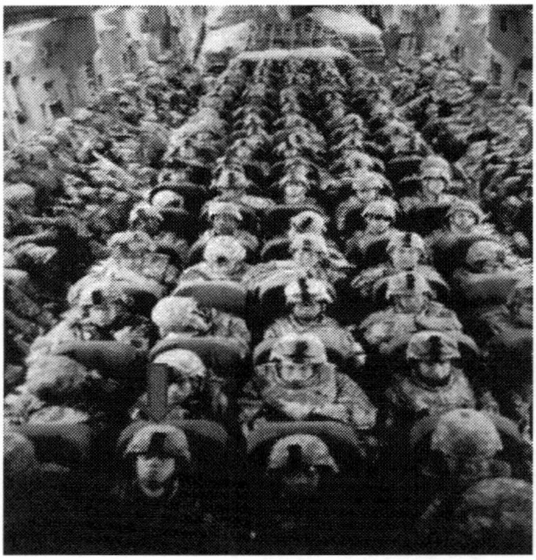

If I thought the flight to Okinawa on a commercial plane was bad, my perspective definitely changed after the C-130 flight to Bagram Airfield. We looked like combat-ready sardines all squished together on a flight that felt like a roller coaster. It was common practice for aviators to perform flight maneuvers before landing to avoid enemy fire, making it feel like one's blood pressure was constantly fluctuating.

Not every medical combat advisor was destined to go to the same place. Some were assigned to Kabul, others to Mazar-i-Sharif and Herat. Assignments were made randomly, and mine led to Camp Stone in Herat, an ancient city with a rich culture and history that dates back more than two millennia. Our training at Fort Polk had taught us that the mission of the medical combat advisor was to "win the hearts and minds" of the Afghan people. That meant mentoring the Afghan National Army (ANA) staff at the Herat Military Regional Hospital on Camp Zafar.

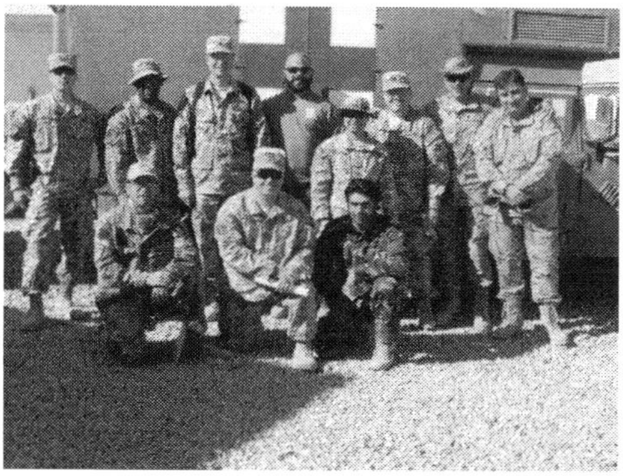

The regional hospital was relatively small, with only fifty beds, and mainly focused on treating ANA, Afghan National Police (ANP), and local civilians. The most common injuries were gunshot wounds and those caused by IED blasts and vehicle rollovers. As the only perioperative advisor in Herat, my role consisted of mentoring and coaching surgeons and nurses in the OR.

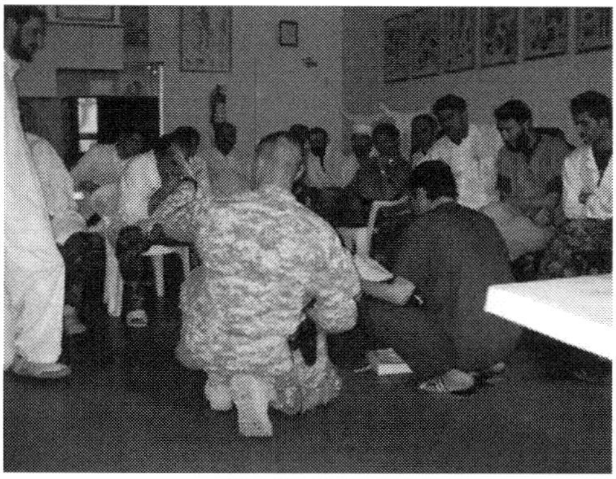

A typical day for a medical combat advisor in Herat began with a meeting first thing in the morning in the Joint Medical Operation Cell (JMOC and our headquarters) to discuss the plan for the day. The biggest risk we encountered each day was the half-mile walk from JMOC to the hospital. The Afghan base where the hospital was located was also a boot camp training site for the ANA and ANP. To mitigate the risk, we would walk in groups of two, locked and loaded with M9 pistols. Physicians, nurses, hospital administrators, and hospital corpsmen alike commuted together as a team and watched each other's backs.

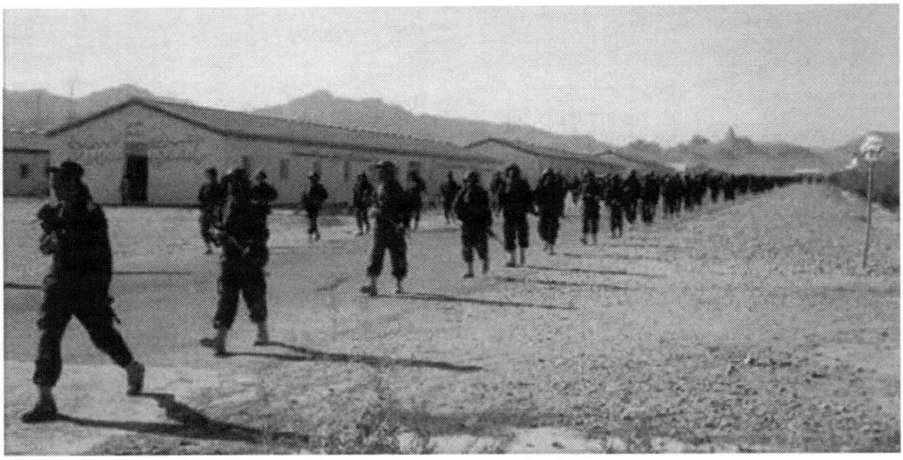

Just like when I learned some Japanese, I had to master phrases I could use to help build rapport with the Afghan hospital staff. Conversational phrases like *salam alaikum* (hello, God be with you), *wa alaikum salam* (God be with you as well), *chetor asti?* (how are you?), *khoob astum tashakor* (I am well, thank you), *wa shoma?* (how about you?), *khoob* (well), *familat khoob ast?* (how is your family?), *familam khoob ast, tashakor* (my family is well, thank you), *chai menoshi?* (would you like some tea?), and *lutfan bale* (yes, please) became part of my everyday vocabulary. Family is at the core of Afghan culture, so many conversations revolve around family matters.

Walking into that OR for the first time was eye-opening. Anesthesia was used sparingly, and the sounds of patients in agony were often heard in the surgical suite. The perioperative practice standards we followed back home went out the window in Herat. It was not unusual to see surgeons working without sterile gloves, picking contaminated surgical instruments up off the floor and placing them back on the surgical back table, delaying surgery to drink *chai* and eat *naan* (I would often be reminded that *inshallah*, meaning that "if God wills," then the situation would turn out just fine regardless of the delay of care), and even bringing patients into the OR without first confirming the procedure that needed to be performed. There was no universal protocol in place to safeguard patient safety. The universal protocol checklist that gets ingrained in perioperative nurse training is a safety measure that was enacted in the U.S. in 2004 in response to the wrong site, wrong patient, and wrong procedure sentinel events.

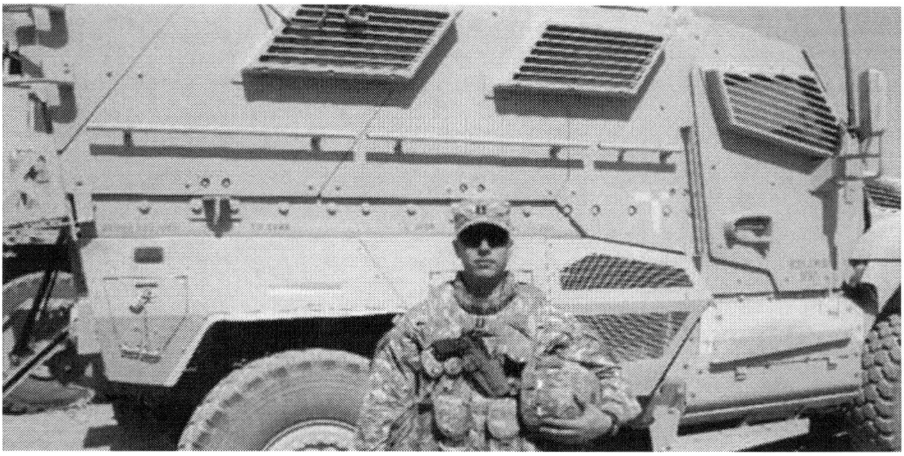

During that time frame, the incidence of wrong site procedures performed in the U.S. was about forty per week. I couldn't have imagined what those statistics looked like in Afghanistan, considering the absence of safety protocols. It's such a simple concept consisting of three basic actions: preoperative verification, marking the operative site, and performing a surgical time-out. I knew very well that I didn't stand a chance at changing their perspective on *inshallah*, but maybe I could help them develop and implement some safety measures. So, I proposed the idea of creating the first Afghan universal protocol checklist, an effort that ended up becoming a success due to the Afghan OR team's commitment to making it work. People often think it takes grandiose ideas and large budgets to make positive change, but this is one example of how impactful change can be influenced without those things.

The return to Okinawa dwarfed any other long flight I had ever been on. Rather than flying east from Afghanistan to Okinawa (3,378 miles), I flew west through the rest of Asia, Europe, North America, and finally back to Japan

(13,564 miles). I had never been so eager to return to the island that had once upon a time made me feel trapped. I was simply grateful to be alive and for the opportunity to have experienced a place I would have never been able to visit had it not been for the Navy. I once again came to appreciate the things that most of us take for granted, like not having to place toilet paper on a toilet seat every day, being able to drive a car without the fear of getting hit by an IED, and not having to walk fifty meters just to take a shower. Nevertheless, I missed home and looked forward to returning to the U.S. after living abroad for three years.

Put It Into Action

Topic/theme	Supporting Evidence	Expected Outcome	Platform
Cultural Competency	VR is efficacious in improving cultural competence in healthcare professionals and has a high user satisfaction rate.[19,20]	Better prepare healthcare professionals for situations requiring high cultural competency. In the military, cross-cultural leadership engagements via VR can equip service members with the communication tools to be influential medical advisors in foreign countries.	BodySwaps Metaverse-based platforms

Teamwork and Safety	Interdisciplinary collaboration and workplace safety can be enhanced through VR education.[21 22]	Reduce communication gaps between healthcare disciplines to improve safety across healthcare. Medical errors are considered the third leading cause of death in the U.S., making initiatives that improve teamwork and safety a top priority.	BodySwaps SimX
Combat Casualty Care	VR addresses operational gaps in the U.S. military and provides greater realism, accessibility, cost-effectiveness, and performance analysis when compared to traditional	Improve operational readiness of U.S. military healthcare professionals in combat casualty care principles, including medical emergencies, chemical, biological, radiological, nuclear, and high explosives (CBRNE),	SimX

	training methods.[23,24,25]	aeromedical evacuation, advanced resuscitative care, and prehospital transport training.	

CHAPTER 6

The Pivot Point

Unlike the Japanese culture, which is known to be calm and soothing, returning to the Mexican culture prevalent in San Diego was overly stimulating. My best friend Jose Medrano and his high school sweetheart Lilli Sandoval welcomed me at the San Diego International Airport and treated me to fish tacos at a taqueria right off H Street and Woodlawn Avenue. The Fito Olivares song "La Gallina" immediately overpowered the serene memories of the Japanese *izakayas*.

The cliché of saying it's a small world gets even more cliché when you're in the military and run into the same people worldwide. At my new assignment, Naval Medical Center San Diego (NMCSD), I would once again be working with my NNMC and Okinawa co-workers Pat Parker and Rob Cuento. They had arrived at NMCSD several months before me, so they were able to help get me all settled in. NMCSD, nicknamed "the Pride of Navy Medicine," had the largest OR in the DoD, averaging 1,000 surgical cases per month. NMCSD's main OR was much larger than Okinawa's (eighteen rooms versus four) and benefited from a broader range of surgical specialties, including cardiothoracic, robotics, total joints, pediatric neurosurgery, vascular, plastics, and bariatric. NMCSD managed pretty much all types of surgery with the exception of cases that required the kind of care one found in Level 1 Trauma Centers, such as car crashes, major brain injuries, blunt force trauma, severe burns and falls, and gunshot and stab wounds.

As a lieutenant (LT) competing against sixty-seven other O-3 (meaning they were at the same pay grade as me) NC officers at the command, I knew I would have to step up my game.

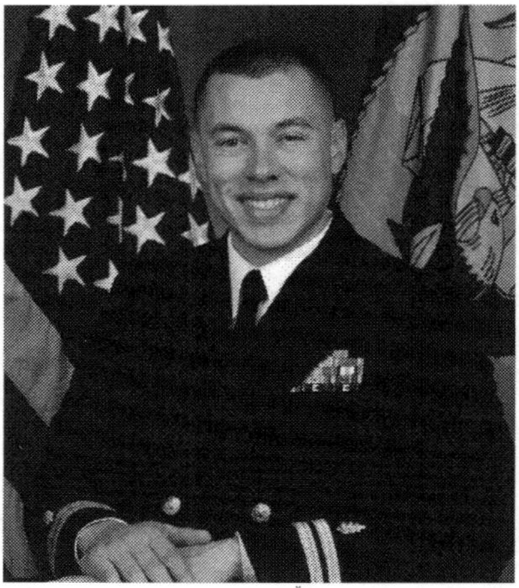

One of the biggest benefits of having started perioperative nursing in a smaller OR was that I could master the basics fairly quickly, and transitioning into the NMCSD main OR was simply a matter of adding extra layers of knowledge and skills to what I already knew. I compare this to making a bean and cheese taco. You only need a flour tortilla, refried beans, and some cheese. But, if you add some ground beef, lettuce, tomato, and some salsa to the mix, you've got a "supreme taco." Constructivism, which is essentially building onto what one already knows, is a core theoretical element for gaining proficiency in the clinical setting. Within a few months of arriving at NMCSD, I was selected to serve as the weekend main OR clinical coordinator, a position that would prepare me well for what was yet to come: another deployment to Afghanistan.

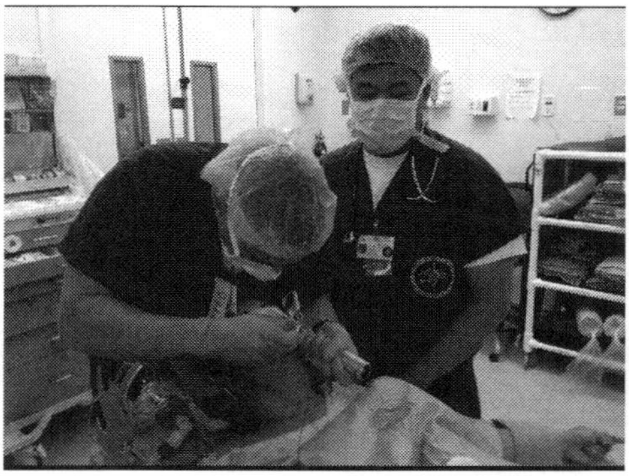

I hadn't given up on my aspirations to become a CRNA, but the eligibility requirements for the program had changed. The OR no longer qualified as a "critical care" setting, meaning I would have to invest countless off-duty hours working in the ICU to fulfill the one-year critical care requirement. Demands at work made this very difficult, so I opened myself up to other options. To climb the ladder in the OR, your business savvy must be just as sharp as your clinical acumen. For this reason, I considered applying to business school under the Duty Under Instruction (DUINS) program. The purpose of DUINS is to provide naval officers with an opportunity to meet critical education and training needs. In the NC, DUINS options typically include doctor of nursing practice, master of science (MS) in nursing, Naval Postgraduate School, post-master certifications, nursing research (PhD), business school, and various other training and fellowship opportunities. The master of business administration (MBA) degree was the only DUINS option for NC officers who wished to continue working in the perioperative setting. It is not what I originally had in mind, but it sounded interesting, and I figured it was worth a shot for the sake of my professional growth.

I was once told that it is not a good idea to earn more than one degree from the same university because it stagnates diversification, so I decided to apply to one of the other great Texas academic institutions: Texas A&M. It was close to home and the program at Mays Business School scored well in overall rankings. Prior to traveling to College Station for my interview, I read the book *The Best Business Schools' Admissions Secrets* by Chioma Isiadinso to gain insight into what the admissions board would be looking for. The section that talked about simply being yourself is what stood out to me the most. That shouldn't be too hard, right? Well, on the day of the interview, I sat in front of a panel alongside five other business school candidates. The first interviewer kicked it off by asking, "Dagoberto, my first question is, what does your name mean?"

I probably considered about a hundred different, appropriate responses to the question for a second, but of course, being who I am—like Isiadinso had recommended in his book—prompted me to respond with, "It means Mexican Brown Bear."

I expected to hear a few chuckles but received none. She then proceeded with a follow-up question. "Well, Mexican Brown Bear, can you please break it down for me?"

I said, "*Dago* means Brown Bear, and when you add the *berto* at the end, it makes it *Mexican Brown Bear.*"

I knew right then and there that my interview had gone south very quickly. I didn't leave College Station with the same motivation I had on the way there. On my flight back to San Diego, I thought that maybe I should just stick to being a clinician for as long as possible. As a perioperative NC officer, this would likely slow down my momentum toward another rank promotion.

I always thought it was good practice to undergo a career development assessment anytime I found myself at a crossroads, whether that meant considering separating from military service, a change in specialty, or if I simply couldn't decide what to do next from a professional standpoint. I wanted to excel in my career, but I knew that being a worker bee in the OR would only get me so far. I was convinced after my MBA interview that business would not be the best thing for me at that particular moment, but I could only think of two other paths I could take at this point: separate from military service to pursue my dream of going to medical school or explore other viable DUINS options. To figure out a solution, I requested a career development board with two officers I highly respected: LCDR Carlin Callaway and LCDR Joseph Hacinas.

After explaining my situation, they both agreed that separating from active duty service would be unwise, considering how much time I had already invested in the Navy. I had been in for thirteen years at that point. The CRNA specialty was a long shot due to the amount of off-duty hours I would need to invest simply to meet eligibility. But then they mentioned a nursing specialty that I hadn't considered before because of how poorly utilized it had been in the past: Clinical Nurse Specialist (CNS).

In this specialty, my job would be to identify clinical problems and then fix them by implementing evidence-based practices. It all sounded pretty straightforward, and I could stick with clinical work while taking on a leadership position. But it was LCDR Ron DeLeon who really convinced me that this was the ideal path for me. CNSs were unique in that they had the flexibility to allocate as much time as they wanted to direct patient care and other administrative tasks. It was like a combination of different nursing roles: clinician, consultant, leader, educator, and researcher. I remember reflecting on my nursing career during this time.

All of my mentors up to this point had been CNSs: LT Tracy Isaac, LCDR Andrea Petrovanie, LCDR Carlin Calloway, LCDR Joseph Hacinas, LCDR David Crumbley, CDR Sarah Martin, CDR Dan Marino, CDR Candy Simmons, and CAPT Brenda Baker. Indeed, this seemed more and more like the right path. So, I decided to test the waters by applying to the University of San Diego Hahn School of Nursing and scheduled a school interview with Dr. Ann M. Mayo. I was committed to never again referencing the "Mexican Brown Bear" during a school interview, so it all went very well. It was now only a matter of submitting an application for the DUINS program; however, that plan was temporarily derailed when I received orders to deploy to Afghanistan for another round, this time to Kandahar.

Ironically, the military has always had limited opportunities for trauma training within its own healthcare system. Only Brooke Army Medical Center (BAMC) in San Antonio has earned the distinction of becoming a Level 1 Trauma Center. However, sending all DoD healthcare professionals to train there is unfeasible. To overcome the challenge of sustaining clinical competencies in trauma, the DoD has established military-civilian partnerships with many different trauma centers around the country, such as Los Angeles General Medical Center, Stroger Hospital of Cook County, University Hospitals Cleveland Medical Center, and Penn Medicine. The Kandahar mission required real-life trauma training as a prerequisite, so I participated in the Navy Trauma Training Center (NTTC) program in Los Angeles in 2013 along with the rest of the healthcare team that was selected to deploy: surgeons, critical care providers, anesthesiologists, CRNAs, nurses (critical care, emergency, and perioperative), and hospital corpsmen.

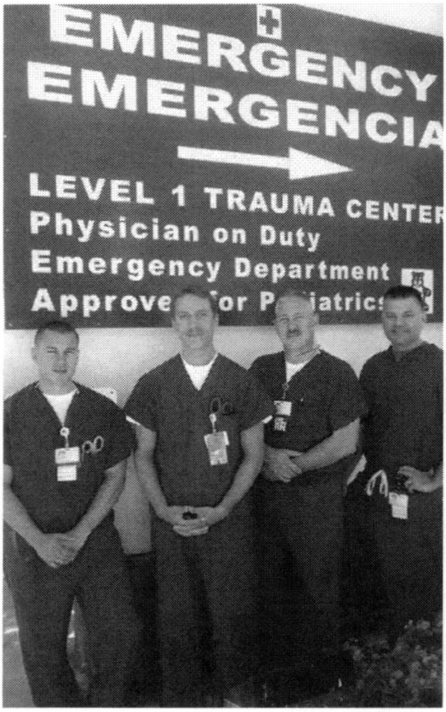

During the intense thirty-day training period, the teams participated in various learning activities, including didactic, skills workshops, trauma simulations, and clinical rotations in the ER, ICU, and OR. It was just enough to get us all in the right mindset to foster teamwork in our respective specialties. Upon completing the training, the NMCSD cohort briefly returned to San Diego to bid our family and friends farewell one last time before heading back to the Middle East.

LCDR Jay Zulueta, an experienced NMCSD perioperative RN and a good friend, was slated to become my roommate while in Kandahar. Jay and I became "peas and carrots" like Forrest and Bubba in *Forrest Gump*. We realized that it was going to be a long deployment when we were shaken up by a mortar attack on our very first night in Kandahar. We laugh about it now, but that night, we found ourselves sheltered in our barracks, lying on the floor in our underwear (we were about to snooze after the long trip). I recall us staring at each other and asking, "What the heck do we do?" These types of experiences form a special bond like no other can. In a sense, one comes to terms with the possibility of death and becomes willing to die for a teammate, regardless of nationality, race, or ethnicity. I couldn't have asked for a better sidekick, and Jay's expertise in trauma and meticulousness made the perfect recipe for success at the NATO Role III Multinational Medical Unit (also known as the combat hospital). It was established in 2005 as part of an

International Security Assistance Force (ISAF) mission, which was then supported by the United Kingdom, the Netherlands, Denmark, Australia, the United States, and Canada. By the time I deployed there in 2013, the hospital had already been turned over to the U.S. Navy and relocated a few hundred feet away from its original site to a high-tech hospital that was 70,000 square feet and rocket-resistant.

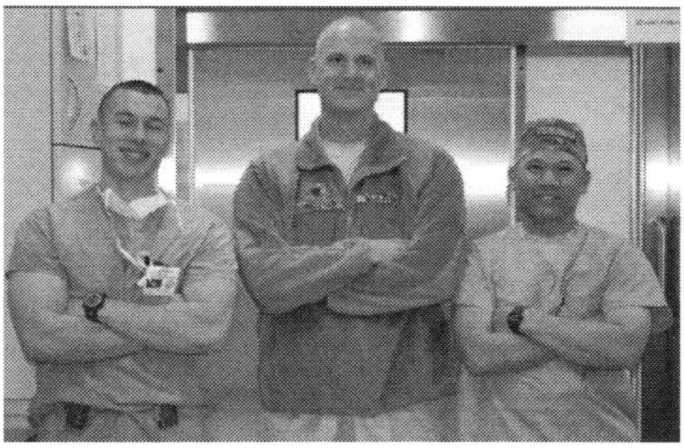

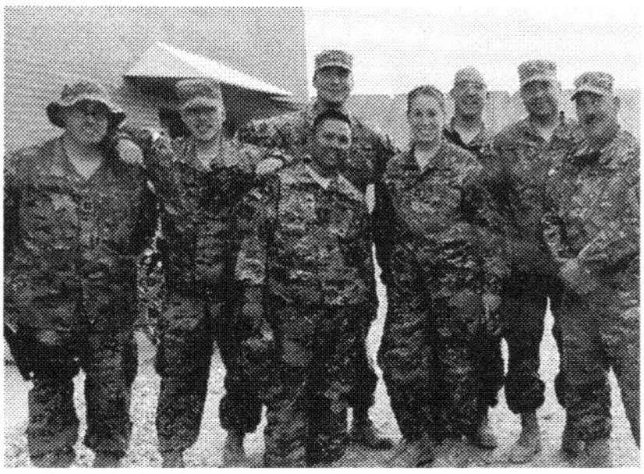

At about my two-month mark in Kandahar, the trauma director, who turned out to be Dr. Travis Polk (the same surgeon who taught me how to properly tuck a patient's arms for laparoscopic surgery in Okinawa), asked me to go on a special trip to Camp Bastion Hospital to learn how to use point-of-care technology called ROTEM (rotational thromboelastometry) from the British. ROTEM falls under the umbrella of viscoelastic measurement studies (viscous, as in a material's resistance to flow, and elastic, or the ability of a material to return to its original state after being stretched), qualities which are useful in examining real-time formation of blood clots. I had never heard of ROTEM, much less knew what it was for, but I agreed to go. Dr. Polk described ROTEM as a technology that could help improve outcomes related to trauma-induced coagulopathy (excessive bleeding or clotting in trauma). Dr. Sean Birmingham, a laboratory technician, and I caught a flight from Kandahar to Camp Bastion. Our arrival felt unreal. The sky looked red, and everything was covered in dust. For a second, we thought we might have been flown to planet Mars. There was no one at the airport to receive us, so we ended up hitching bus rides and asking for directions until we finally made it to the hospital.

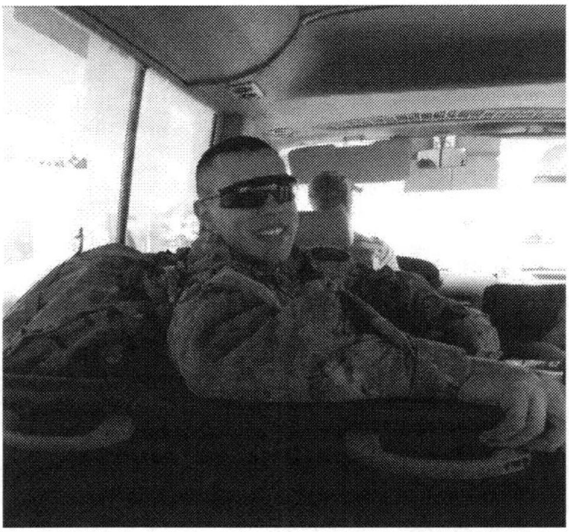

Once we arrived, we connected with Lt. Col. Elizabeth Mann-Salinas (no relation to me, but ironically married to a Salinas from the Laredo area), who taught me everything I needed to know about ROTEM from diagnostic testing and troubleshooting to maintaining an effective quality control process. I spent a week in the ER, OR, and ICU running ROTEM tests. It quickly became an obsession that led me to further explore the pathophysiology behind trauma. In essence, the main objective behind implementing ROTEM in Kandahar was to have a tool that could expeditiously help us identify coagulopathies and treat them with precision. If the results indicated low platelets, we gave platelets; if the results showed low clotting factors, we gave fresh frozen plasma (FFP). If the results indicated low fibrinogen, we gave patients cryoprecipitate; if the results showed clot breakdown, we gave tranexamic acid. By default, I became the ROTEM expert and assumed responsibility for educating and training the rest of the OR team.

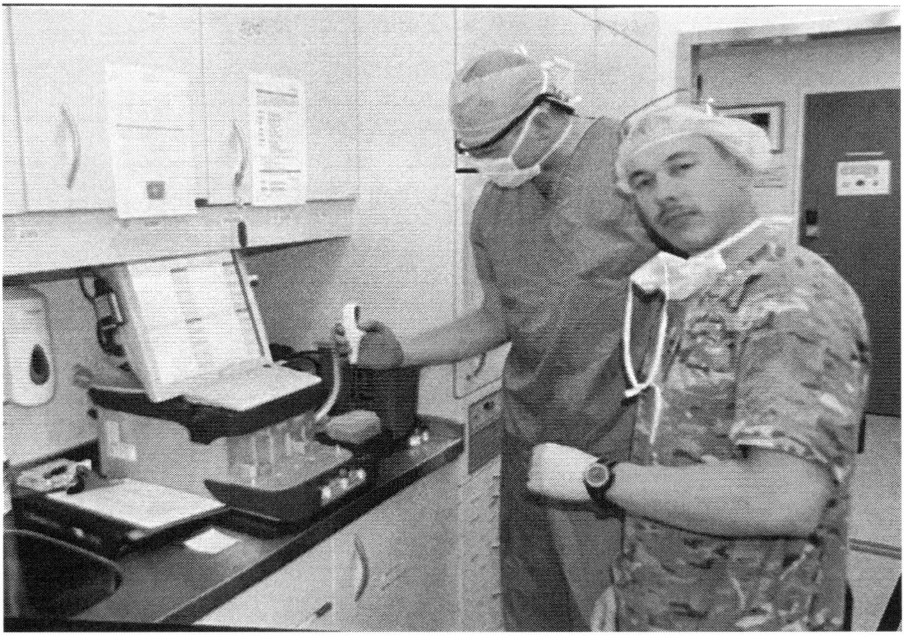

Our time in Kandahar went by quickly. Between caring for the wounded in the OR, managing the ROTEM program, and playing chess with Slovaks (I lost every game), the deployment soon ended.

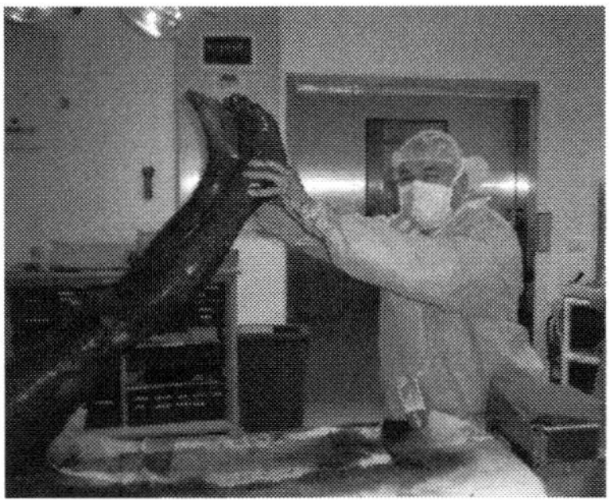

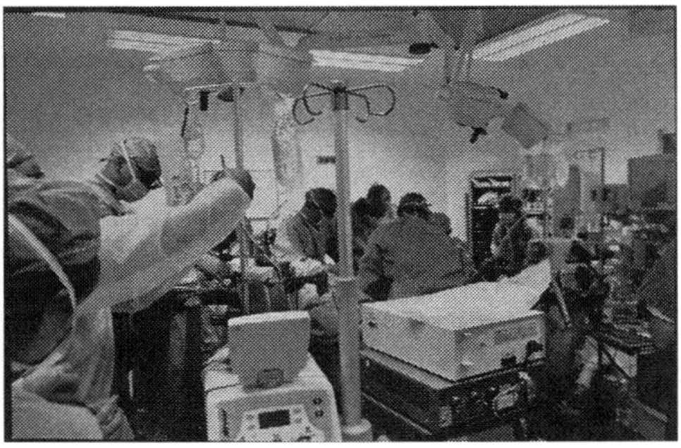

Returning to San Diego was bittersweet for me. On the one hand, I found out that I would be promoted to the rank of lieutenant commander and attend graduate school through the DUINS program: adult-gerontology CNS option. On the other hand, my personal life had spiraled out of control due to an unexpected divorce after eight years of marriage. I had never felt so numb in my life. Nevertheless, I needed to continue pushing forward because defeat was not a word I had in my vocabulary. Enrolling in the University of San Diego CNS program was no longer viable because the last thing I wanted to do was remain in San Diego. So, I Googled the best CNS programs in the U.S. and came across the University of Pennsylvania—a program that is now obsolete.

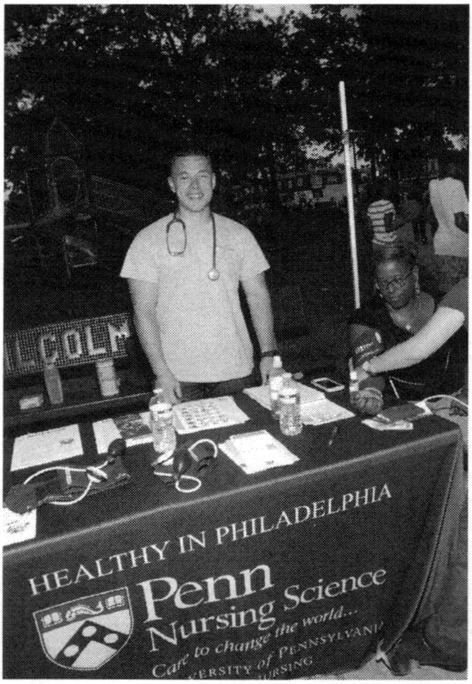

In August 2014, I hit the road in a U-haul with my uniforms, civilian clothing, two Tim Cantor paintings (he's a local painter in San Diego), and an HP printer. That's it! The 2,695 miles between San Diego and Philadelphia were enough to help me clear my mind and focus on what awaited me. The decision to move to Philadelphia to heal mentally was a pivotal point in my life. Rather than doing the right thing and seeking professional mental health services when I needed them the most, I indulged in alcohol and academia. I felt like the two of those went together. Drinking made me want to write, and writing made me want to drink. The CNS program at UPenn was nothing short of impressive. Between the Hospital of the University of Pennsylvania (HUP), Jefferson Hospital, Jefferson Methodist Hospital, and Pennsylvania Hospital, I was able to work with some of the best CNSs the country has to offer.

People like Amy Moore, Sitha Dy, Anne Muller, and Ruth Lebet were instrumental to my growth as a CNS. However, nothing can fully prepare you for the CNS world. It simply takes time and experience to get the hang of things.

As a capstone project, I felt compelled to tell the world about the potential benefits of ROTEM technology. Exploring the topic was perfect because not only did it involve a clear clinical problem (poor patient outcomes related to trauma-induced coagulopathies), but there was plenty of research to support its implementation. It was at this point that I fell in love with writing. In a way, writing became therapeutic because it removed me from reality. I often compare it to playing chess because there are so many different ways to achieve the same goal. There is not necessarily a right or wrong decision, just a better way. I still remember Sitha at HUP drilling me so I'd get more specific when writing abstracts.

"But why, Dago? Why is ROTEM important?"

"Because it saves lives, Sitha."

"But *how*?"

"Well, you run a test, and the software tells you whether or not there's coagulopathy present."

"And why does that matter?"

"It matters because you can then effectively treat the trauma or surgical patient with the appropriate blood product."

"There you go, Dago! That's it! ROTEM helps guide proper blood product administration during trauma and surgical resuscitation. Good job!"

Simply saying that ROTEM saves lives was not incorrect, but there was a better way of describing it. Thanks to Amy, Sitha, Anne, and Ruth, my first manuscript submission was accepted for publication by the *Association of Perioperative Registered Nurses (AORN)*[26] in 2016 and was subsequently selected as the article of the year. This achievement was a good way to start off my first assignment as a CNS at Naval Hospital Jacksonville (NH Jax).

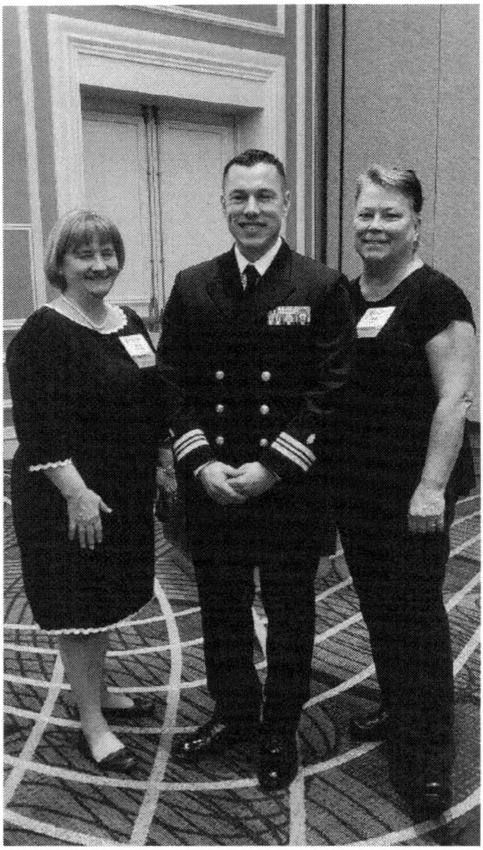

Put It Into Action

Topic/theme	Supporting Evidence	Expected Outcome	Platform
Surgical Education	VR provides a safe and realistic environment to further develop surgical skills and confidence.[27,28,29,30]	Augment current modalities used in surgical education to improve outcomes in the	PrecisionOS OssoVR FundamentalVR VantariVR

		perioperative environment.	
Trauma Care	Clinical skills, empathy, and teamwork in trauma settings can be enhanced through VR.[31,32,33,34]	Offer additional trauma training opportunities that are realistic and accessible. Military paraprofessionals, such as Navy HMs, Army medics, and Air Force technicians, could gain valuable trauma skills that could benefit them in combat environments.	SimX VRPatients
Critical Care	VR can serve as an adjunct to traditional training modalities in critical care environments and improve medical experiences for adult and	Improved simulation experiences for a variety of critical care skills, including central venous line placement, cardiopulmonary resuscitation, extracorporeal	Metaverse-based platforms SimX

	pediatric patients, relatives, and providers.[35,36,37]	membrane oxygenation device management, endotracheal intubation, and management of ectopic tachycardia, low cardiac output, and acute respiratory failure in pediatric patients.	
Laboratory Environment	VR provides effective immersive learning experiences in laboratory environments that are difficult to access physically.[38,39]	Provide learners with additional opportunities to learn about different laboratory environments and equipment. For example, to facilitate their adoption in trauma settings, military medical providers could be taught about viscoelastic studies, such as ROTEM.	Facilitate VR

CHAPTER 7

The Patient, Staff, and Organization

The main takeaway from most CNS graduate programs is that they operate as subject-matter experts at different levels within the healthcare system: patient, staff, and organization. But what exactly does that mean? In the military, I often compared these different levels or "spheres of influence" to the three levels of warfare: tactical (nursing department), operational (nursing directorate), and strategic (hospital and beyond). In simple terms, one must be able to liaise between the three by working directly with patients, leading and educating nursing staff, and implementing best practices through research and policy. Historically, the CNS specialty has been difficult to conceptualize because it can be difficult to quantify the work produced. The specialty dates back to the 1960s and is one of the four advanced practice nursing designations: the CRNA, the nurse practitioner, the midwife, and the CNS. The other specialties are much easier to describe and quantify.

For example, a CRNA administers anesthesia, and their work can be quantified by the number of procedures completed. A nurse practitioner is considered a provider, and their work can be quantified by the number of patients seen. A midwife is a birth specialist, and their work can be quantified by the number of newborns delivered. But how in the world can one accurately measure the work of a CNS when fluctuating between patients, staff, and organizations?

I worked at NH Jax from 2016 to 2019. It's a community-size hospital in Jacksonville that supports the U.S. Navy's third-largest fleet and serves as many as 163,000 beneficiaries through partnerships with local hospitals and physicians in the TRICARE network.

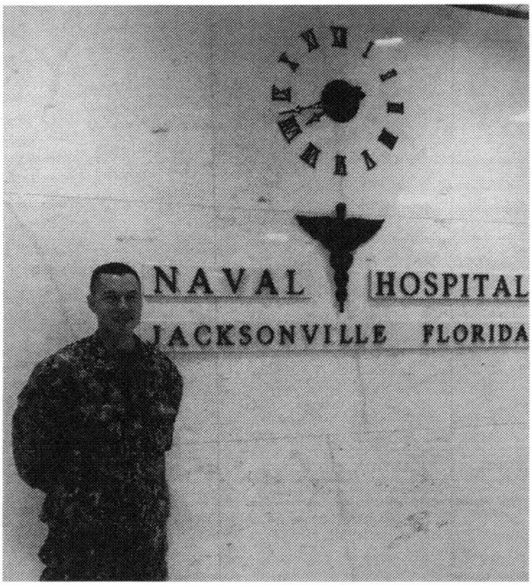

Although the hospital felt small compared to others I had worked in, it had a unique vibe, great leadership, and a strong foothold in Navy Medicine. NH Jax had been selected as the pilot site for the navy's administrative transition to the Defense Health Agency, a transition that has since transformed military healthcare operations. However, whether that is good or bad, only time will tell. Upon my arrival, I met with my chief nurse executive, CAPT Jeffery Johnson, a leader who I later came to appreciate as one of the best nursing leaders I have ever worked with. He was also a CNS, so he knew where and how to move his chess pieces. A CNS is analogous to a knight on an empty chessboard. A knight can theoretically land on every square regardless of where it started and end up on its original square without touching the same square more than once (this is known as the knight's tour). No other piece really describes a CNS. Pawns are too one-dimensional, bishops are too limited, rooks have a long range but are too predictable; we are not typically queens or kings unless we choose the nurse executive path. Knights are just right; our day-to-day activities are unpredictable, and we have the potential to move into any space when we calculate our moves carefully.

In our meeting, CAPT Johnson gave me three tasks: improve clinical practices in MSU, refine RN and HM competency processes throughout the hospital, and implement a nursing grand rounds initiative to promote professional development. But first, I was asked to learn how to place peripherally inserted central catheters (PICCs) to augment the hospital's vascular access team. All I said was, "Roger that, sir, I will do my best."

My PICC training experience went well, considering our limited resources. Katie Davitt, a seasoned ICU RN and nurse educator, was in charge of the vascular access program; however, she only had about a year left before her retirement and needed to train her replacement quickly. Honestly, there weren't too many RNs to choose from who would have the flexibility to drop whatever they were doing and step in. So, Katie decided to get me trained. It was important for NH Jax to have an in-house PICC RN available; otherwise, PICC insertions would get outsourced and become a financial burden to the hospital.

Katie didn't waste any time and signed me up for a computer-based PICC insertion course that I had fifteen days to complete before moving on to the hands-on portion of the training. Anecdotally, this training pathway is fairly typical. After submitting my certificate of completion to Katie, she scheduled a one-on-one training session to teach me ultrasound. She covered all the basics of the equipment and then had me practice several times on a Jell-O mold (made by the NH Jax Education and Training Department) that contained three plastic tubes inside: small, medium, and large. Practicing on a Jell-O mold was an inexpensive way to learn the motor skills associated with ultrasound-guided needle insertions. Next, Katie introduced me to the PICC kit and its contents. I remember unfolding the fenestrated drape and then struggling to put it back in its original position (I am the kind of guy who has a hard time putting inflatable mattresses back in the box). After getting a feel for what the procedure should look like (with the help of YouTube videos), I joined Katie to observe a PICC line insertion. NH Jax only had one or two PICC insertion requests per week, so I needed to take advantage of any opportunity to observe the entire process from start to finish when I could. Unlike starting an IV, inserting a PICC involves many more steps and requires more caution, especially with the sterile technique. Fortunately, my

OR experience made the sterile technique component a bit easier. Nevertheless, there was still a very steep learning curve. Katie made the procedure look too easy.

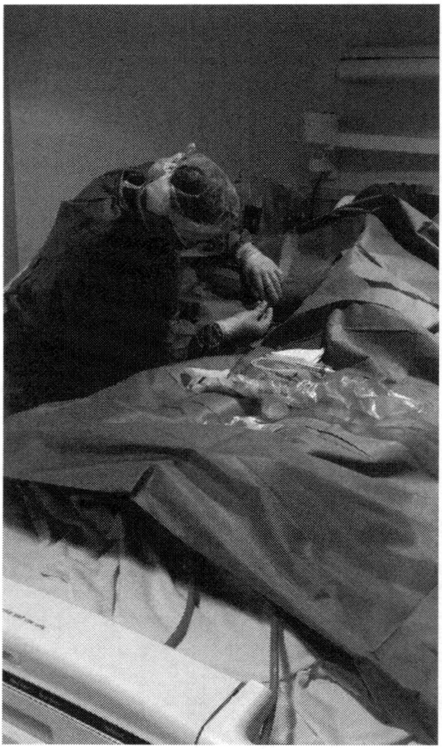

Katie called my office phone the following week and asked, "Are you ready?" There was a PICC order, and she decided it was a good time to have me scrub in. My heart started pounding instantly. I re-watched one of the YouTube videos I had found just to refresh my mind. It all made sense in my head, but would I remember all the steps once I entered the room? Katie arrived right before the video ended to take me to where the procedure would be done. This experience reminded me of my first IV attempt on USS Valley Forge; I was so preoccupied with the little things that I butchered the more critical steps of the procedure itself. Check the patient's labs, get informed consent, confirm the length measurement, give the patient some local anesthetic, remove the dilator before advancing the catheter, locate the antimicrobial disc, and confirm the patient's arm circumference: it's not that I didn't already know these steps, I just felt that I hadn't practiced them enough to make the procedure go as smoothly as possible. They call this cognitive overload. There were simply too many small details to process, making it difficult to focus on other obvious things. In retrospect, having more realistic, accessible practice sessions could have helped lessen my cognitive load in this case.

After I completed the procedure, Katie took about fifteen minutes to evaluate my performance. My ultrasound technique was spot-on, but I really needed to work on all the other critical components of PICC placement. She stressed, "You can teach a monkey how to obtain vascular access, but the critical thinking part…" In the end, Katie reassured me that I would be okay next time as long as I addressed the things we discussed. A funny fact about me is that I learned to type as many as ninety words per minute as a teenager by mentally typing words and doing the finger motions. Using this same technique, I used mental repetition to rehearse every single step of PICC insertion, from obtaining informed consent and checking labs to sequentially performing the insertion and completing my documentation. I became obsessed with mastering it all in my head so I'd get it right the next time I physically performed the procedure.

Meanwhile, I began working on the tasks that CAPT Johnson had assigned me by exercising what I learned in the UPenn CNS program. There are many different types of implementation or change management models, but here is more or less how I learned to tackle CNS projects.

1. **Identify the problem.** What is wrong with the current method? Why change? Who are the stakeholders?

2. **Collect information related to the problem.** Quantify the problem by collecting more information about it.

3. **Perform a literature search.** Find out what has already been published about the identified problem. Chances are that this problem has already occurred elsewhere.

4. **Organize your findings.** Create a table of synthesis to outline the findings of each published piece of literature that you found. In your table, include the source, the publication date, the type of evidence presented, methodology, findings, strengths and limitations, relevance to your topic, the citation, and any comments or notes you come up with.

5. **Evaluate the findings.** Figure out if the findings were positive or negative. Are they indeed relevant to your problem? Would it be realistic to implement this information in your clinical setting?

6. **Implement.** In coordination with the relevant stakeholders, implement evidence-based practices and establish a method for measuring the outcome.

7. **Disseminate your findings.** Share the results with department staff, clinical practice committees, and external entities (conferences, publications, webinars, etc.).

8. **Monitor the new process.** Implementation is easy, but sustaining the new process can be challenging. Maintain a good process for continual, positive change!

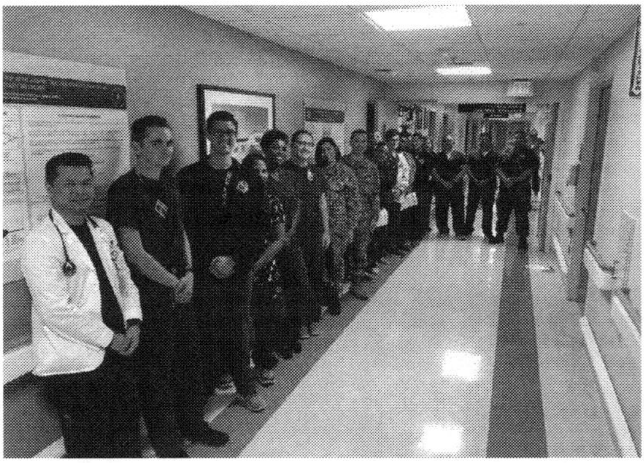

The task of improving clinical practices for the MSU was so broad that it allowed for autonomy in deciding what exactly needed to be done. It was a perfect time to meet my staff (the General William Bester way), conduct a strengths, weaknesses, opportunities, and threats (SWOT) analysis, and identify stakeholders along the way. In simple terms, my objectives were to first discover the problem, find a solution, implement the solution, and sustain it. The MSU was a twenty-bed telemetry medical-surgical unit that admitted patients ranging from thirty days of age to geriatrics. Out of forty-eight staff members, 69% were military staff members with less than three years of clinical experience, so it quickly became evident that the civilian staff kept the

MSU afloat. I know that military personnel tend to gravitate toward other military co-workers, but establishing a strong, professional relationship with civilian staff is fundamental to success.

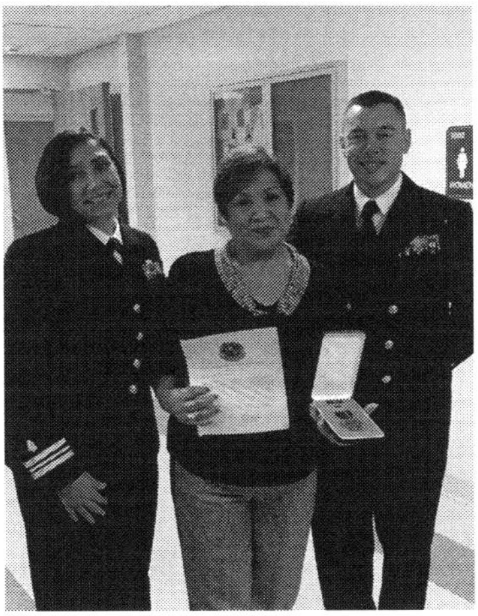

While military service members rotate in and out of different commands and deploy, civilians remain constant. My biggest advice to military leaders is to treat their civilians well, and in turn, they will make you look good. If there is anyone who really understood that concept well at NH Jax, it was my department head, LCDR Candy Anderson.

She took care of the administrative tasks for the MSU while I handled the clinical side. Together, we got things done. After examining our SWOT findings and diving into our patient safety reports, we determined that the source of MSU's clinical challenges was related to how our staff was onboarded. Onboarding was unstructured and disorganized, and the challenge was further compounded by the frequent turnover of military staff members (both RNs and HMs). Furthermore, the MSU didn't have a well-established education and training process for novice RNs and HMs. One day, during our morning coffee and brainstorming routine, LCDR Anderson and I decided to standardize our educational delivery methods by leveraging a competency-based online platform called Elsevier Clinical Skills and creating a simulation

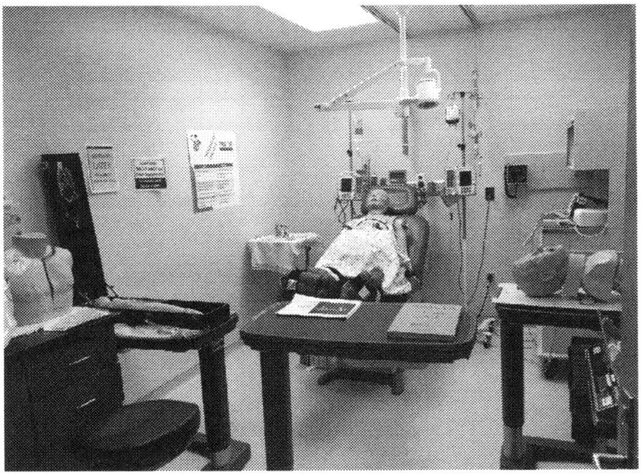

lab to implement all the necessary training into practice. This was not a high-tech lab; it was simply a space that was not being utilized appropriately at the time. In collaboration with the hospital's education and training department, we added a full-size manikin, zoll defibrillator, chest tube drainage system, PCA, IV and feeding pumps, electrocardiogram machine, Foley catheter with bladder irrigation set, central line dressing change station, nasogastric tube with suction, and blood product administration set.

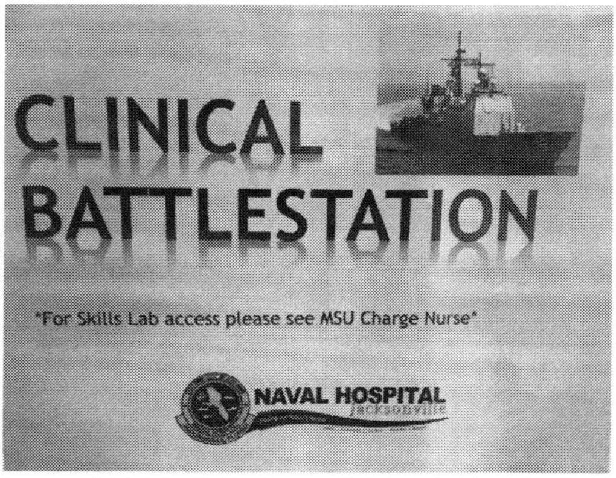

To engage the staff in the process, we created clinical scenario development teams to help set up realistic MSU scenarios. To top it all off, we named the simulation lab "Clinical Battlestations" and added a photo of USS Valley Forge on the door sign to honor the ship, which taught me the value of repetition and realism in training. The MSU's clinical practices were improved by standardizing the onboarding process and fostering better clinical skills practice through a simulation lab.

Through this process, we also realized that the hospital faced similar challenges. Clinical competencies were not standardized and outdated, meaning that many clinical decisions were being made without the support of current, evidence-based recommendations. Using the MSU as a blueprint for clinical practice, I proposed via the Nursing Practice Committee to standardize clinical competencies throughout the hospital. For example, there was no reason why an RN working in the ICU should do a central line dressing change any differently than an RN working on a medical-surgical floor. An RN working in the ER should start a peripheral IV the same way an RN working in labor and delivery would. Studies I had previously read indicated that variations in clinical practice led to poor quality of care and increased costs, so it was prudent of us to streamline our KSAs and standard operating procedures.

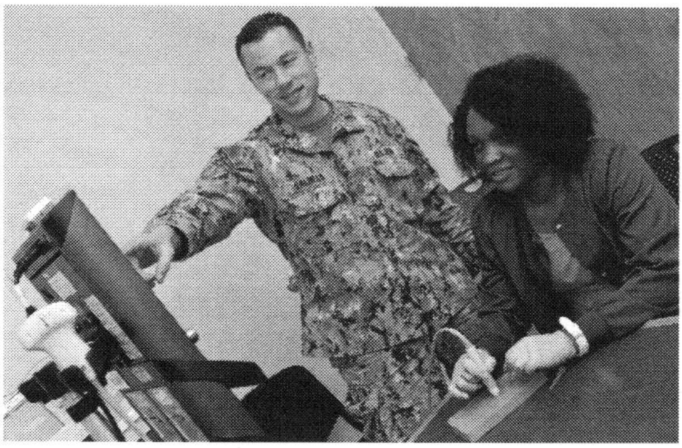

One of our projects aimed to improve first-time IV insertion and blood draw success rates. During that time, it was typical for difficult venous access (DVA) patients to get stuck more than five times in a row for IVs and lab draws. We prioritized this project because DVA patients would often receive a PICC placement order due to a high number of failed attempts to insert an IV, which would then open up a different can of worms. In the literature, first-time success rates for IV insertions are reported as 76%–91% and 53%–75.6% for adult and pediatric populations, respectively. To put this into perspective, about 70%–80% of hospitalized adult patients will receive an IV, and one out of five of those hospitalized patients will experience multiple IV or blood draw attempts. It is no surprise that IV insertion is considered the most commonly performed invasive procedure in the hospital setting. Coincidentally, I had already completed my PICC insertion certification, so the idea of piloting an ultrasound-guided peripheral intravenous (USGPIV) initiative was one of the first ways I thought of to improve first-time IV success rates.

Following the implementation model I outlined earlier, here's what the process looked like.

- **Identify the problem.** Too many IV insertions and blood draw failure rates lead to more PICC insertions, which opens the door to more infections associated with central lines.

- **Collect information related to the problem.** DVA patients were getting stuck at least five times for IV insertion, resulting in delays in their treatments and diagnoses.

- **Perform a literature search.** Studies showed that USGPIV practices were superior to traditional palpation methods in obtaining first-time access in DVA patients. Evidence also suggested that it was a skill that was acceptable to teach to technicians, such as HMs.

- **Organize your findings.** I created a table to organize details from all the supporting evidence I had found.

- **Evaluate the findings.** The evidence for implementing a USGPIV protocol looked very favorable, so I created a presentation for the Nursing Practice Committee. Not only was it approved, but funds were allocated to purchase a dedicated ultrasound machine for the MSU. I give LCDR Anderson all the credit for making this purchase happen.

- **Implement.** We designed a blended USGPIV skills competency program. Elsevier Clinical Skills was leveraged to standardize the knowledge component, and then we scheduled one-on-one instruction sessions that would utilize silicone molds.

- **Disseminate your findings.** In collaboration with other stakeholders, we published our findings in *MEDSURG Nursing.*[40]

- **Monitor the new process.** A standard operating procedure outlining USGPIV practices in the MSU was created to sustain its implementation even beyond my tenure at NH Jax.

To address the third task that CAPT Johnson had assigned me (implementing a nursing grand rounds initiative), I followed the same exact format. First, I needed to identify the problem and ultimately establish a process for sustainable change.

Here's the information structured into a checklist format:

- **Identify the Problem.** Recognize the lack of a hospital-wide interdisciplinary grand rounds program at NH Jax, which hindered staff learning opportunities.
- **Collect Information Related to the Problem.** Conduct an educational needs assessment to understand staff engagement preferences. Identify interest in learning about high-risk, low-volume scenarios through case studies correlating with the hospital's patient safety reports.
- **Perform a Literature Search.** Research the history and effectiveness of nursing grand rounds, focusing on their impact on knowledge, self-confidence, and teamwork.
- **Organize Your Findings.** Create a table of evidence to organize all supporting data found on the topic.
- **Evaluate the Findings.** Assess resource needs, proposing a bi-monthly presentation schedule. Align the initiative with the Navy NC campaign for professional development.
- **Implement.** Launch the nursing grand rounds with a presentation on ROTEM and coagulopathy management in combat casualty care. Collaborate with ENS Carlos Robles to provide mentorship and peer learning in a non-judgmental setting.
- **Disseminate Your Findings.** Expand the grand rounds virtually to naval medical facilities and a local civilian hospital. Reflect on the

success driven by interdisciplinary teamwork and partnerships. Publish results in the American Journal of Nursing.

- **Monitor the New Process.** Include nursing grand rounds in the Nursing Practice Committee's monthly agenda. Conduct a twelve-month post-implementation survey to evaluate the initiative's impact on clinical knowledge, research discussion, professional development, teamwork, and partnerships.

It is a common saying that "time flies when you're having fun," and yes, it does. It wasn't long before I received orders to transfer to my next and final duty station: Navy Medicine Training Support Center (NMTSC) in San Antonio. It was atypical for a navy commander to get orders to instructor school, but my situation was a bit unique. I received transfer orders as an O-4, but my promotion to the next rank was unexpectedly sped up. In 2019, the Navy implemented meritorious promotions for the top two performing officers of their respective selection boards, which would allow immediate promotion regardless of seniority. That year, I ranked second out of thirty-four NC officers selected for the pay grade of O-5. CAPT (Ret) Brenda Baker (my career-long mentor) promoted me on my final day in Jacksonville in front of my MSU family.

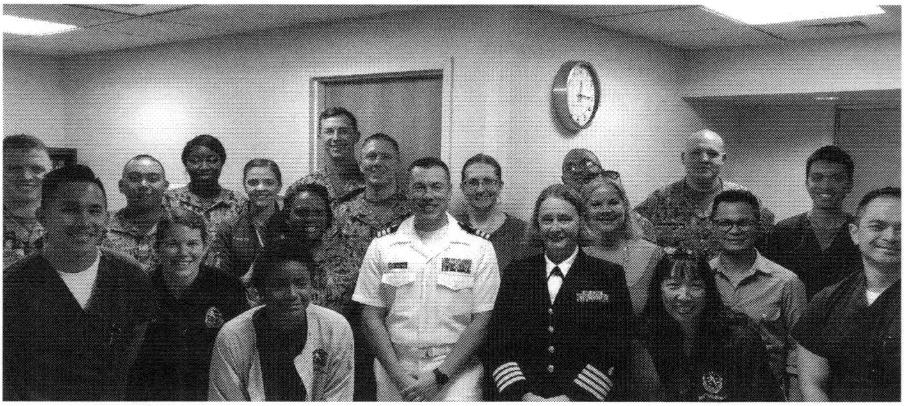

Ironically, I would end my naval career teaching at the school I always dreamed of attending as a young enlisted sailor. I never did become an HM, but this was my one opportunity to make an impact on the rating that I had learned to respect like no other.

Put It Into Action

Topic	Supporting Evidence	Expected Outcome	Platform
Vascular Access	VR can effectively augment traditional training modalities in vascular access by providing a realistic environment that improves familiarity with procedural workflows.[42,43,44]	Increase confidence and clinical skills in novice PICC inserters and provide a standardized method for evaluating annual skills competencies in more experienced providers. VR could further complement current vascular access education and training curriculums by providing learners with more holistic opportunities for practice.	SimX

Grand Rounds	Compared to traditional grand rounds delivery methods, VR offers improved visualization of clinical findings, radiologic imaging, and labs.[45,46,47]	An enhanced grand rounds learning experience that can be scaled globally.	Metaverse-based platforms

CHAPTER 8

Corpsman Up!

Becoming a Navy NC officer early in my military career was a blessing. However, part of me wished that I had experienced the HM journey. I knew that I couldn't change my past in terms of how I joined the Navy, but I could at least make an impact on the HM rate by sharpening its education and training practices.

Since its creation in 1898, the HM rate has become the most decorated job in the military: twenty-two Medals of Honor, 179 Navy Crosses, 959 Silver Stars, and more than 1,600 Bronze Stars. A total of twenty naval ships have been named after HMs, in addition to the three main administrative and academic buildings that comprise NMTSC: HM3 John T. Fralish, HM2 Jaime S. Jaenke, and HM3 Christopher Alan Anderson. NMTSC serves as the navy's central command, overseeing administrative and operational functions for personnel and students enrolled in medical programs in the San Antonio area. With a dynamic population made up primarily of new boot camp graduates and fleet returnees, the command typically hosts more than 2,500 students and 500 instructors and support personnel.

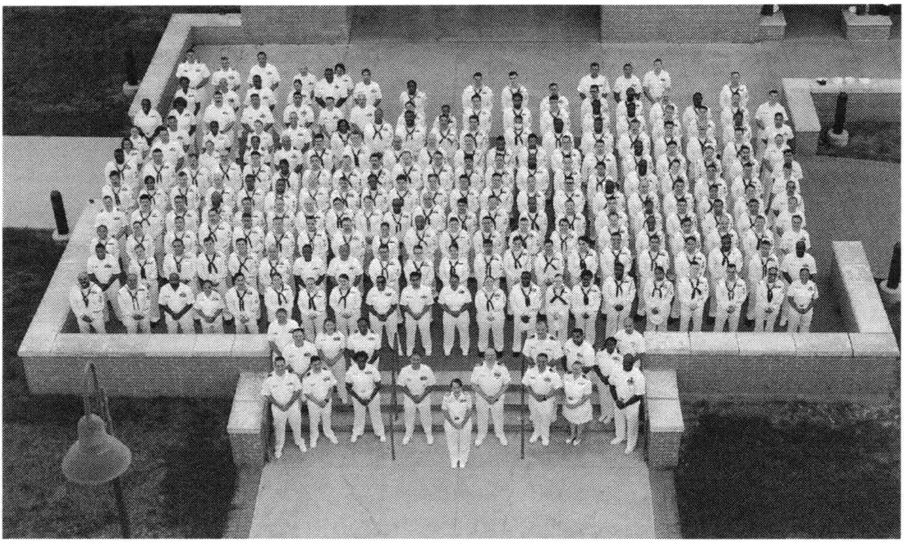

In 2019, I decided to accept orders to NMTSC primarily due to my desire to address the declining clinical skills I had observed at NH Jax. On average, the MSU received two or three new HMs each month, and I became familiar with their baseline skills, which I believed required fine-tuning. This issue, like any other, had a root cause: Hospital Corpsman Basic (HCB), also known as HM "A" School. There was no one to blame, but the deterioration of clinical skills in HM graduates correlated with a significant curricular change at HCB during that time frame.

The HM and Air Force technician curricula had merged, only to see the two programs split a few years later. There was too much change. HM "A" School is where HM students learn basic life support, medical terminology, anatomy & physiology, pre-hospital care, and inpatient and outpatient procedures. So, rather than complain about the issue, it was now my turn to do something about it by shifting gears from clinician to instructor. Many would argue that taking on this assignment as a newly promoted O-5 would be a career killer due to the limited high-impact leadership opportunities available, but, at the end of the day, promotion was not the motivating factor behind my decision to instruct at HM "A" School. It was more personal than that. I have since been asked many times to share the keys to success as a naval officer.

It's very simple: don't do things for the sake of a promotion. Do things because you are passionate about them, and everything else will fall into place." I think this idea also applies to many other aspects of life. Don't get a job you don't like just because it pays more. Don't pick a major in college that only interests you because it offers more high-paying opportunities post-graduation. Don't choose Kashi cereal over Cap'n Crunch just because it's healthier (maybe this is not a good example).

I had no idea what to expect at NMTSC, but I was confident that I could figure things out just like I had before through an implementation model. How hard could that be? It was just a matter of identifying the problem and working my way through it, right? Well, not quite.

- **Identify the problem.** The voice of the customer (Navy Medicine and its affiliates) indicated that HM "A" School graduates lagged behind in entry-level KSAs. In other words, they lacked current knowledge, skills performance, and attitude development.

- **Collect information related to the problem.** Much of the instructional content found in the student handbooks was outdated. To make matters worse, clinical practicums were permanently taken out of the course curriculum.

- **Perform a literature search.** Studies show that evidence-based curriculums in the health profession are fundamental to ensuring that students graduate with current knowledge and are prepared to deliver safe, quality patient care. Healthcare systems rely on the knowledge and skills of new graduates to practice safely and call on academic institutions to advocate for practicums that promote KSA proficiency in clinical settings.

- **Organize your findings.** I created a table of evidence to organize details from all the supporting evidence I had found.

- **Evaluate the findings.** The evidence for supporting an HM "A" School curriculum revision and defending the need to keep clinical rotations available was prevalent. It was clear that change was needed to satisfy the customer's needs (Navy Medicine and its affiliates).

- **Implement.** This phase was *not* completed. During this phase, I realized that the idea of transforming how HMs were educated and trained was much more complex than I had initially thought. I had been at NMTSC for a few months and still didn't fully understand the interplay of all the different commands involved. First, we had our mother ship, Naval Medical Forces Support Command (NMFSC, where the curriculum originated). Next, we had the Medical Education and Training Campus (METC, where the curriculum was maintained), and NMTSC (where instruction took place). To make a major curriculum change, NMTSC would first need to request changes through METC, and then METC would need to make a request to NMFSC. Depending on the nature of the request, this could take several weeks, months, or even years.

- ~~**Disseminate your findings.**~~ Never made it to this phase.

- ~~**Monitor the new process.**~~ Never made it to this phase.

I knew that if I were going to accomplish what I had set my mind on before leaving NH Jax, I would have to take a leap and apply for a position within HM "A" School that would allow me to take the next steps towards change. That was the program director position, a role scheduled to become available in the spring of 2020. Unfortunately, I was not selected for the job. Instead, NMTSC leadership decided that my skills would be better suited for a command position that blended four different roles: compliance officer, executive steering committee sponsor, quality management, and public affairs. I was perplexed by NMTSC's decision to have me handle their compliance program.

However, this was at the top of the priority list due to a scheduled Navy Medical Inspector General (MEDIG) program visit in 2022. MEDIG inspections take place roughly every three years to evaluate a command's effectiveness, capability, and quality in accordance with directives and instructions from the Secretary of the Navy, the Office of the Chief of Naval Operations, and the Bureau of Medicine and Surgery. I had limited experience maintaining a compliance program, but just like anything else, I knew I could find resources to help me navigate these uncharted waters.

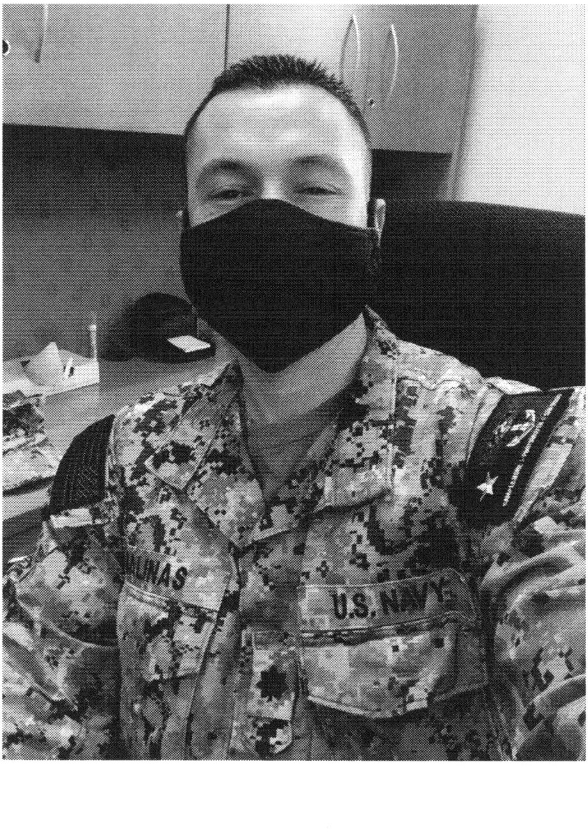

The MEDIG compliance program is structured very much like the U.S. Department of Health and Human Services Office of the Inspector General (OIG). A health compliance program has seven keys: written policies and procedures, a chief compliance officer, education and training, open lines of communication, a discipline policy and follow-up actions, internal or external audits and compliance monitoring, and responses to detected deficiencies. To maintain compliance with this program, I found two actions to be extremely vital in my day-to-day work: maintaining strong communication with program managers and establishing a rigorous internal monitoring and auditing tempo. It was important for me to establish rapport and connect in real-time (not just via email) with the thirty-four MEDIG program managers that we had at the command. The tricky part, however, was maintaining a rigorous internal monitoring and auditing tempo. The command inspection was scheduled within twelve months of my taking on this new job, so we needed to ensure that all programs were in top shape.

Considering we had thirty-four MEDIG programs at the command, I figured conducting twelve audits per month (three per week) would allow me to get a good pulse on every program at least once per quarter. I like to compare preparing for an inspection to training for a marathon. One would be a fool to just get out of bed and run without any training. The key is to be consistent and work in short and long runs every day leading up to the event. The tedious part about internal monitoring and auditing was not meeting with compliance managers but having to track the organization's status manually. Everything was paper-based and in spreadsheets! Here is what the sequence of auditing looked like.

1. Identify the program to be audited.
2. Log into my desktop computer and print a current audit checklist from the MEDIG program home page.
3. Travel to wherever the program manager is located.
4. Conduct the audit and take good notes on the hard copy of the audit checklist.

5. Travel back to my office.
6. Log into my desktop computer and transcribe what I wrote on paper in an electronic version (to keep it all legible).
7. Manually update my compliance MEDIG program spreadsheet.
8. Retain a paper copy of the audit checklist.

It was no wonder my MEDIG compliance officer predecessor was not a fan of internal monitoring and auditing. It was painful then and continues to be so today. Nevertheless, NMTSC's command inspection in 2021 was a huge success, achieving the highest inspection score that Navy Medicine had seen in the past five years. This particular experience inspired the founding of a second company called ComplyDash, which I had the privilege of co-founding with my good friend Karl Larson in August 2023. But that's a story for another book. :)

I never thought I would say it, but after working my first administrative job, I began to miss patient care. Up to this point, I had figured out a way to make it to the O-5 pay grade by doing more patient care than administrative work, but this is rare for a non-provider NC officer. To satisfy my itch to return to the clinical setting after the MEDIG inspection, I shifted my attention to reestablishing a clinical skills program for NMTSC NC officers at BAMC. The DoD's only Level 1 Trauma Center was literally next to our command, so why not take advantage of this great opportunity? I really enjoyed learning advanced vascular access procedures at NH Jax, so I figured I would reach out to the vascular access team at BAMC for an opportunity to brush up on my skills. I hadn't placed a PICC or midline catheter in nearly two years, but I knew that with the right coaching, I could pick up where I left off.

First, I felt it was necessary to enroll in another PICC/midline training certificate program to review the latest research and evidence-based practices. I signed up for a refresher course through CVC Health Care to do so. This company specializes in providing all healthcare professionals with education on the insertion, care, and maintenance of vascular access devices. Overall, I was very impressed with the curriculum and felt that the knowledge and skills aspect of their KSAs were spot-on; however, the attitudes part of the KSA acronym is very difficult to address in traditional training because it requires some form of immersive training, whether that means a real-life or simulated clinical environment.

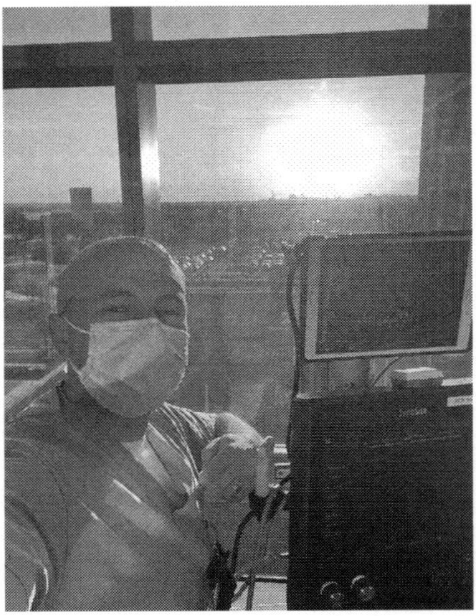

The vascular access team at BAMC was dynamic, with forty years of advanced vascular access experience between Joaquin Polanco, Eloy DeRobles, Lee Demonica, and Rachel Abowd. After completing all my guest provider privileging requirements, I spent numerous hours shadowing each of them to become familiar with their insertion protocols. I had learned how to place PICCs at NH Jax the traditional way, which meant not trimming them to appropriate lengths, nicking the skin with the scalpel before inserting the introducer, and confirming tip placement at the end of the procedure with an X-ray. The BAMC team practiced differently and helped each other remain evidence-based. The orientation experience made me feel like an old dog trying to learn new tricks and further confirmed my need to refine a few procedural steps in my PICC insertion process. These are some of the changes I adopted to improve my technique.

1. I learned how to measure the PICC length more accurately to trim to an exact length rather than coil up the PICC's external length.
2. I learned how to avoid nicking the skin before inserting the introducer by using the introducer tip as an atraumatic way to dilate my way into the vessel.

3. I learned how to use electrocardiogram (ECG) tip locator technology to reduce the number of X-rays needed to confirm final PICC placement.

I embraced these new practices, but the learning process could have gone much smoother and faster had I had access to training modalities that allowed for repeated practice.

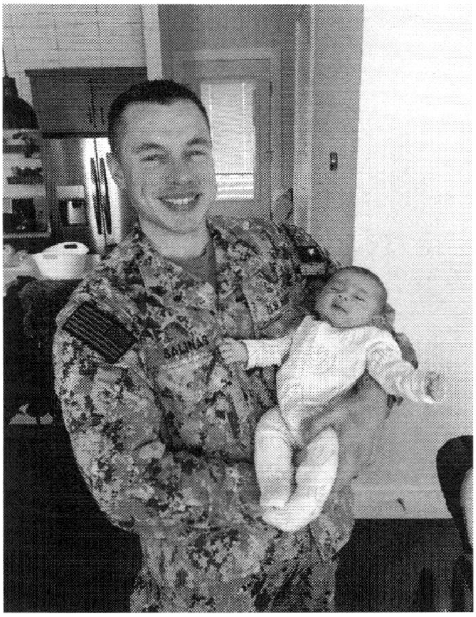

I don't recall sharing this with anyone during this time other than my wife, Scarlet, but part of me felt unfulfilled and frustrated with the bureaucracy of government work. I remember someone telling me long ago that I would know when it was time to leave the military. For the first time in twenty years, I was starting to get the feeling that my service was coming to an end. Everything from logging in to computers to making strategic decisions felt slower and more cumbersome.

The frightening part, however, was the thought of eventually deploying again and leaving my family behind, especially now that our daughter Adelina had joined us. When Scarlet and I started dating in 2017, she made it clear that she was very family-oriented and preferred to have a more stable life. When we married in 2018, I vowed to prioritize our family no matter what. It would be unwise for me to put myself in the same position I had been in before, so I made the decision to retire.

I needed an exit strategy but did not want to leave without first giving back to the HM community. Rather than spending my final months at

NMTSC headquarters, I requested to return to HM "A" School to find fulfillment in teaching again.

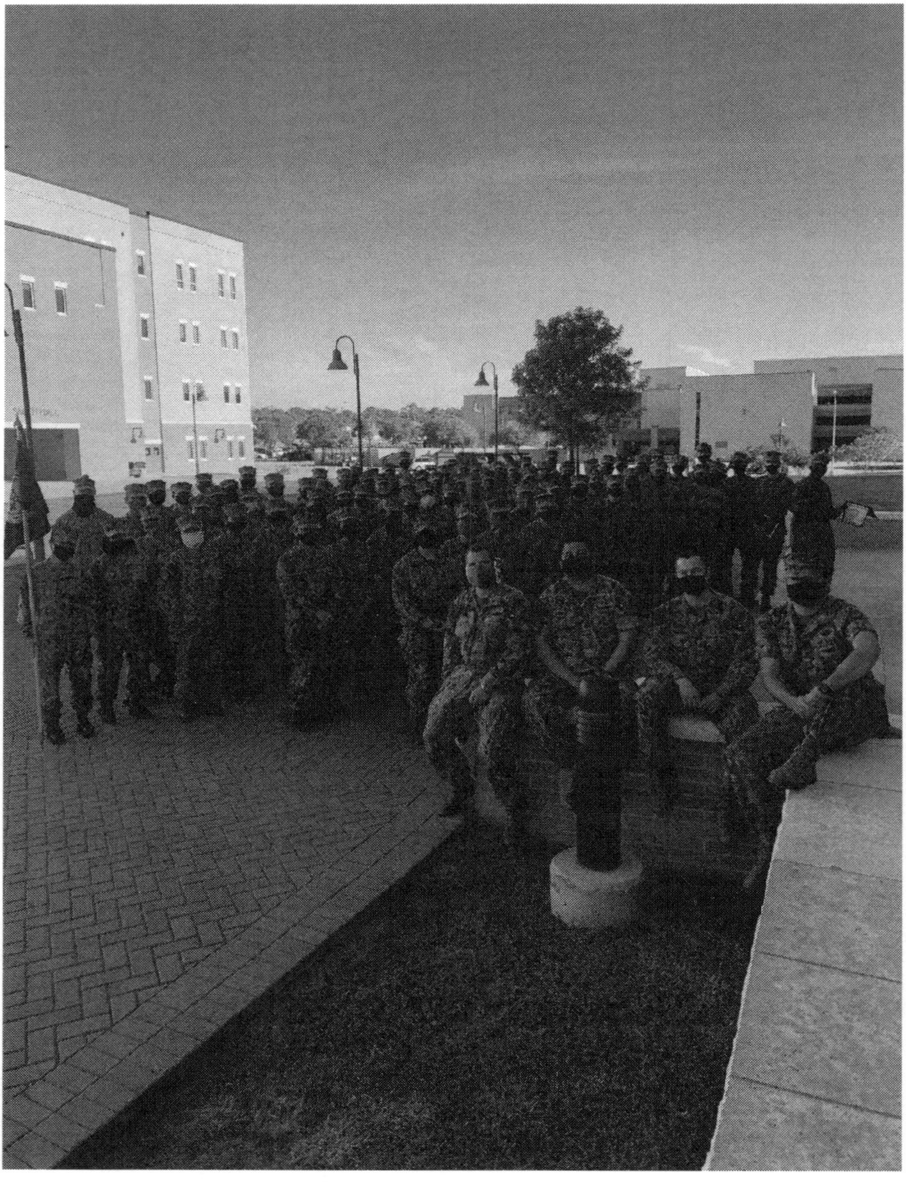

Some people may call it a coincidence, while others may call it fate, but I believe my return to HM "A" School was in God's plan. One of our instructors, LT Bilma Diaz, was exploring the idea of submitting a TriService Nursing Research Program (TSNRP) grant proposal to pilot a VR simulator in the Tactical Combat Casualty Care (TCCC) course. She had an excellent vision for the initiative she wanted to propose but needed assistance getting her ideas on paper and connecting with the appropriate stakeholders. I had already learned my lesson about academic stakeholders in 2020 when I hit a roadblock in my attempt to reshape education and training at HM "A" School, so my goal was to not let LT Diaz experience the same thing. I gladly accepted her request to serve as her project mentor, and we got to work.

Prior to getting involved with the TCCC VR education project, I knew little about VR. How did it compare to traditional training? What were the benefits? It was enlightening to read about how VR was becoming more popular in healthcare, specifically in medical and nursing education. I became convinced that VR had the potential to become the new training platform for planning complex operations. If you think about it, that's pretty much anything in healthcare. Unfortunately, patient safety and quality usually take a big hit when things become more complex. How would we neutralize the growing potential for human error as healthcare continues to evolve in complexity? I will say that it won't be by doing things the same way we've always done them. Healthcare professionals are responsible for engaging and accepting innovations that support positive patient outcomes. Over the course of twelve weeks, LT Diaz was able to demonstrate that VR modalities in TCCC training could be both effective and scalable, as evidenced by two outcomes: acceleration of learning (which would also mean less time spent on training) and the improvement of simulated survival rates of trauma patients compared to past performance.

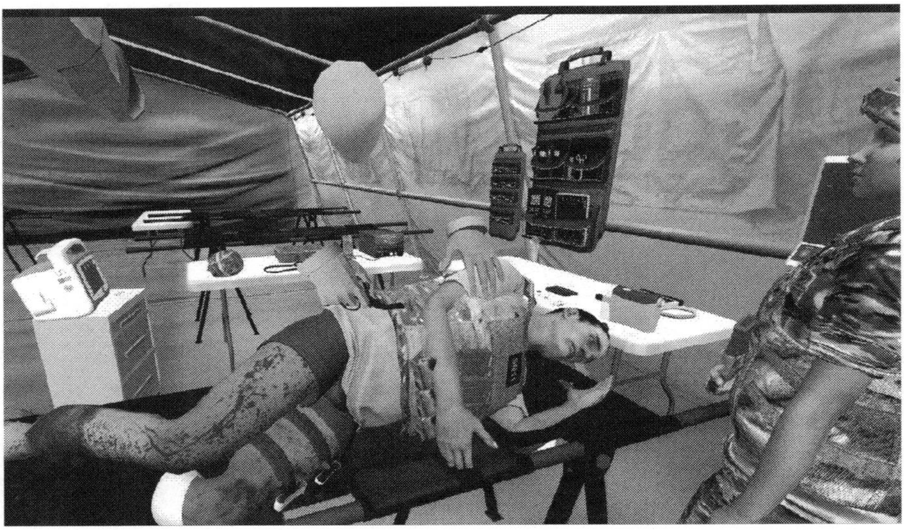

(Photo courtesy of SimX, used with permission)

The cost of the pilot is also worth mentioning. With a small grant of only $10,000, LT Diaz managed to operate VR clinical simulations for a class of forty HM students. It only took several wireless headsets costing $250 each plus a software subscription to get the job done. And then it hit me: *Why not leverage VR technology to help educate and train more vascular access specialists?* Wouldn't an immersive VR environment be more suitable for learning PICC insertion than mentally rehearsing all the steps? From personal experience, opportunities for PICC insertion practice are minimal. What happens to the novice RN who just took a four-hour course and is now expected to perform a PICC insertion on an actual patient? Normally, preceptorship is available at their respective facility, but why not provide additional, more accessible training to boost their confidence further?

I decided to dedicate all my time and effort to exploring innovative ways to reshape vascular access education and training. This also confirmed my decision to retire after twenty-three years of service and pursue entrepreneurial opportunities that I knew would provide solutions to the challenges I experienced throughout my naval career. I officially retired on April 30, 2023.

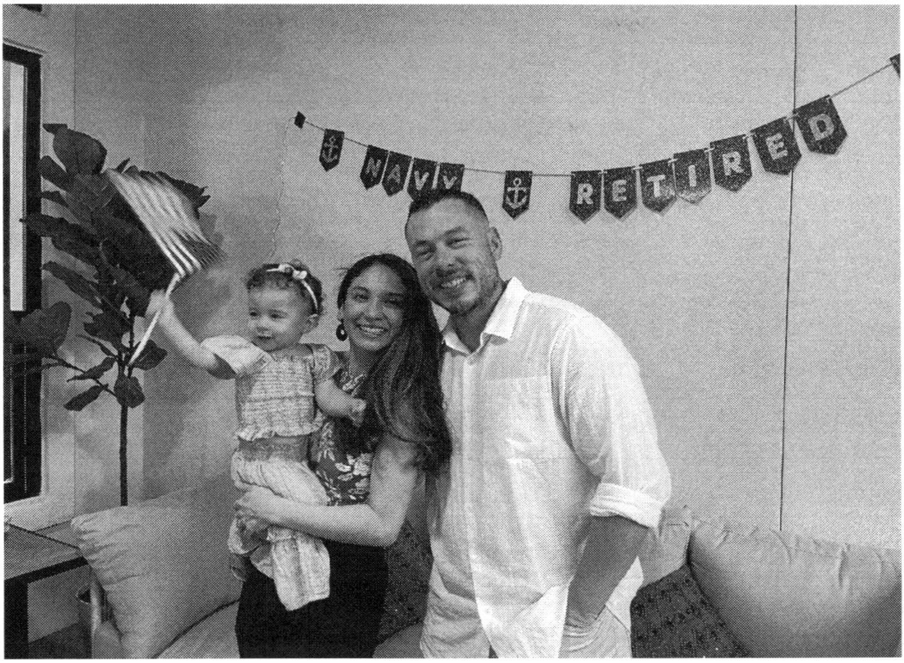

Put It Into Action

Topic/Theme	Supporting Evidence	Expected Outcome	Platform
Anatomy Education	VR may offer an alternative to traditional anatomy education by reducing the ethical concerns associated with	Provide solutions to challenges associated with traditional anatomy training, such as safety and ethical concerns	3D Organon GigXR

	cadaver dissections. Further, VR allows for customization and repeatability of exercises that may not be possible in traditional methods. The gold standard, however, is a combination of both traditional and VR.[48,49]	and limited repeatability.	
Basic Life Support	VR can effectively be used to augment traditional basic life support courses.[50,51]	In combination with traditional methods, VR could further support knowledge acquisition and clinical performance in healthcare professionals.	SimX VRPatients
Pre-hospital Training	Stress management, decision-making, and	Enhance the preparedness of pre-hospital healthcare	ENGAGE SimX

	self-confidence in pre-hospital personnel can be fine-tuned through VR.[52,53,54,55]	professionals by providing a cost-effective method to practice complex triage scenarios repeatedly.	
Compliance Management	Compliance Software as a Service (SaaS) streamlines regulatory adherence by automating the tracking, documentation, and reporting processes, reducing the risk of non-compliance penalties. It also enhances organizational efficiency by providing real-time updates and centralized access to compliance-related data,	Reduction in regulatory fines and legal issues, as the software ensures all requirements are meticulously tracked and met. Also, companies can expect improved operational efficiency and enhanced reputation, as automated compliance processes free up resources and demonstrate a commitment to adhering to industry standards.	*Not a VR platform* ComplyDash

	facilitating better decision-making and resource allocation.[56,57]		

CHAPTER 9

Do Something About It

How many times have any of us complained about the inefficiencies of our work environment? I know I have countless times. When we are faced with these types of situations, we have one of four choices: do nothing about it and just keep to the status quo, remain in that same environment but try to do something to improve it, jump ship and look for other opportunities, or leave but do something about it through alternate means. I chose the latter.

The more I reflected on my life experiences, the more potential solutions I could identify for ordinary, everyday challenges. Initially, I considered introducing VR as a tool to improve how vascular access specialists are educated and trained. But first, I needed to validate whether this was a viable solution. I connected with SimX, one of the world's leading VR medical simulation training platforms designed specifically for nurses, physicians, and first responders. I had no idea if VR training was even available for vascular access, so I needed to connect with a reputable VR medical simulation company that could help me figure that out.

Surprisingly, there was nothing on the market for PICC and midline insertion training. However, SimX offered me the opportunity to partner with them to develop the first PICC/midline insertion simulator. A partnership meant business, so I founded CLINSPEC Solutions, LLC. I consulted with several trusted entities: CVC Health Care owner Mary Smith, PICC Pros owner Joaquin Polanco, Precision Vascular owners Kevin Rogers and Marivic Guzman, and Peak Vascular Access's chief operations officer, Mike Baker. Mary validated the idea from an education and training standpoint; Joaquin and Marivic validated it from a clinical practice viewpoint. Kevin and Mike validated it from a business stance.

Developing a VR simulator for PICC and midline insertions made sense, but my experience with simulation was limited to that of a consumer. To truly bridge my knowledge gap, I felt it would be prudent to learn more about medical simulation from one of the nation's best: MGH Institute of Health Professions (IHP).

I really admire self-taught people who have the patience to take that initiative and make it look like they have been doing something for years. There are good examples of this in my own family. My dad, Dagoberto Sr., learned how to play the piano, violin, guitar, flute, accordion, and saxophone on his own. My mom, Margarita, learned how to use different accounting and financial software tools to manage her logistics company. My sister, Stephany, learned how to make furniture from scratch by watching YouTube videos. Besides learning how to play chess, I haven't learned anything worth bragging about and have primarily relied on formal education or instruction to learn things. I find value in learning the theory before attempting to perform a new skill.

For this reason, I applied to the Health Professions Teaching and Learning post-graduate certificate program at MGH IHP. I considered many different Veteran Affairs-certified programs, but MGH IHP set itself apart through the quality of its faculty and its active engagement with students. In a single semester, I learned things that would have taken me much longer to learn on my own, such as simulation standards and guidelines, pre-briefing and debriefing protocol, simulation template design, and program evaluation. All of these principles, combined with theory and strategies, were instrumental to the overall implementation strategy for VR simulation in PICC/midline insertion.

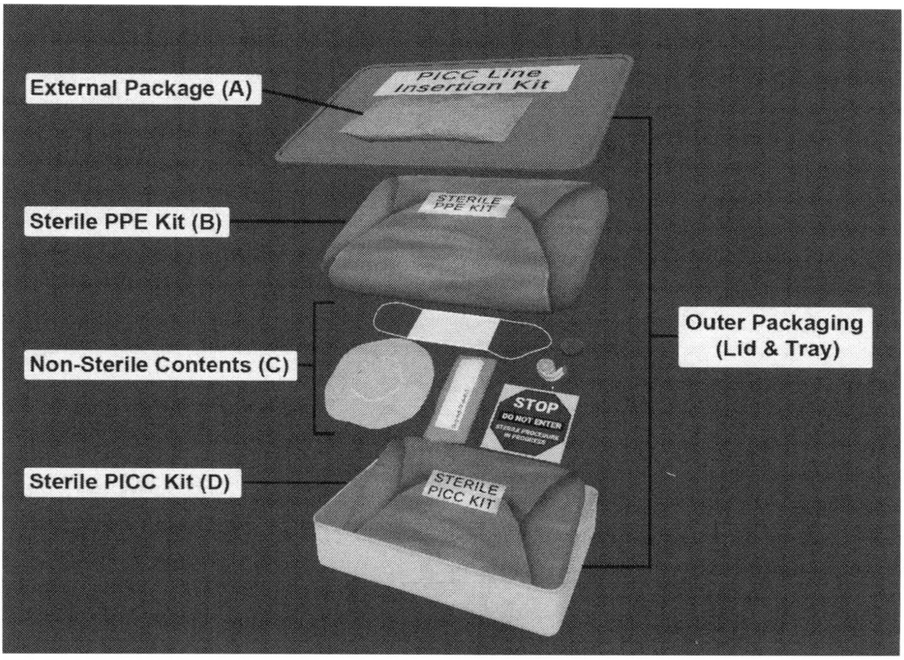

(Photo courtesy of SimX, used with permission)

The golden ticket, however, was receiving feedback from various experts on the proposed simulation template. At the beginning of my program, I had no idea what a simulation template was, but Dr. Suzie Kardong-Edgren helped me overcome that obstacle. In health professions, a simulation template serves as a blueprint for educators to ensure that simulations effectively address learning objectives and provide students with a realistic clinical experience.

Here are some must-dos for those of you considering venturing into healthcare simulation.

1. **Familiarize yourself with the Healthcare Simulation Standards of Best Practice.** These standards were developed by the International Nursing Association for Clinical Simulation and Learning and designed to furnish evidence-based recommendations for

simulation education and operations. They provide a roadmap for planning, implementation, and evaluation of simulation scenarios.

2. **Identify a learning theory or a combination of theories that align well with your idea.** For the vascular access VR project, I deferred to the mastery learning theory because it's designed to systematically take a learner from one milestone to another until they've mastered the skill. Plenty of research supports repetition as a means of promoting plasticity in the brain (a form of rewiring your neurons to improve long-term memory).
3. **Operationalize your simulation template.** This means envisioning yourself in a simulation scenario and seeing what needs to occur to meet your program's objectives. Then, put it all on paper like a blueprint or an outline. There are many examples out there that you can reference on MedEdPort.org.
4. **Last but not least, network with stakeholders and experts in the simulation field.** You don't know what you don't know until you connect with others who have already been there and done that.

There are numerous ways to tackle VR implementation in healthcare, but your education and training needs will ultimately dictate your approach. Below is a simplified list of things you and your team should consider when implementing a VR program.

- Figure out what education and training gaps you are attempting to fill.
- Why do these gaps exist? What's missing in your current program?
- Think about supplementing, not replacing, your current education and training modalities.
- Are there any constraints to using VR, such as space or internet connectivity?
- How many learners do you have?
- What does your budget look like? Can you afford the investment?

- Have you considered hiring a consultant to help implement and sustain the practice?

In the case of **vascular access education companies**, here's what implementation could look like.

- Review your customer feedback. Are they 100% satisfied with their hands-on training?
- Think about where VR could fit into your existing curriculum. What does your current training structure look like? Do you perform assessments along the way?
- Does your budget allow for the purchase of headsets and software licenses? Have you explored financial opportunities such as grants, donors, or partnerships?
- Assess your current training space.
- How many learners per PICC/midline course do you have?
- Explore the different VR headsets available and make sure the ones you purchase are wireless and high-quality to decrease the odds of cybersickness.
- What does your IT support and Wi-Fi accessibility look like?
- Commit to learning how to moderate VR to enhance the learning experience. VR medical simulation companies like SimX provide onboarding tutorials.
- Find a consultant to help you implement and sustain your VR practice. CLINSPEC Solutions, LLC is one option, but many other reputable ones are also available.

In the case of a **hospital setting**, here's what implementation could look like.

- Review your annual competency and onboarding education and training procedures. Are there any gaps?
- Assess your current training space.
- How many learners per class do you have?

- Does your budget allow for the purchase of headsets and software licenses? Have you explored financial opportunities such as grants, donors, or partnerships?
- Explore the different VR headsets available and make sure the ones you purchase are wireless and high-quality to decrease the odds of cybersickness.
- Commit to learning how to moderate VR to enhance the learning experience. VR medical simulation companies like SimX provide onboarding tutorials.
- Find a consultant to help you implement and sustain your VR practice. CLINSPEC Solutions, LLC is one option, but there are many other reputable ones available to you.

In the case of an **academic setting**, here's what implementation could look like.

- Review your student feedback. Are they 100% satisfied with their hands-on training?
- Think about where VR could fit into your existing curriculum. What does your current training structure look like? Do you perform assessments along the way?
- Does your budget allow for the purchase of headsets and software licenses? Have you explored financial opportunities such as grants, donors, or partnerships?
- Assess your current training space.
- How many learners per class do you have?
- Explore the different VR headsets available and make sure the ones you purchase are wireless and high-quality to decrease the odds of cybersickness.
- Commit to learning how to moderate VR to enhance the learning experience. VR medical simulation companies like SimX provide onboarding tutorials.

- Find a consultant to help you implement and sustain your VR practice. CLINSPEC Solutions, LLC is one option, but there are many other reputable ones available.

Again, the decision to add VR to your curriculum should be based on your educational needs. Regarding vascular access, I would also reiterate that the goal of using VR is to supplement, not replace, traditional education and training.

Don't judge, but I need to make another *Forrest Gump* reference. As I neared the end of the VR vascular access project for PICC/midline placement, I couldn't help but think of how Forrest Gump ran from coastline to coastline. Once he reached the end of one journey, he pushed his limits and continued to the next challenge. Why would I limit the idea of advocating for VR implementation to just the vascular access specialty? My professional experiences have demonstrated a dire need to enhance traditional education and teaching methods in every aspect of healthcare. It would have been a game changer if VR NICU training existed sixteen years ago when I struggled at NNMC Bethesda.

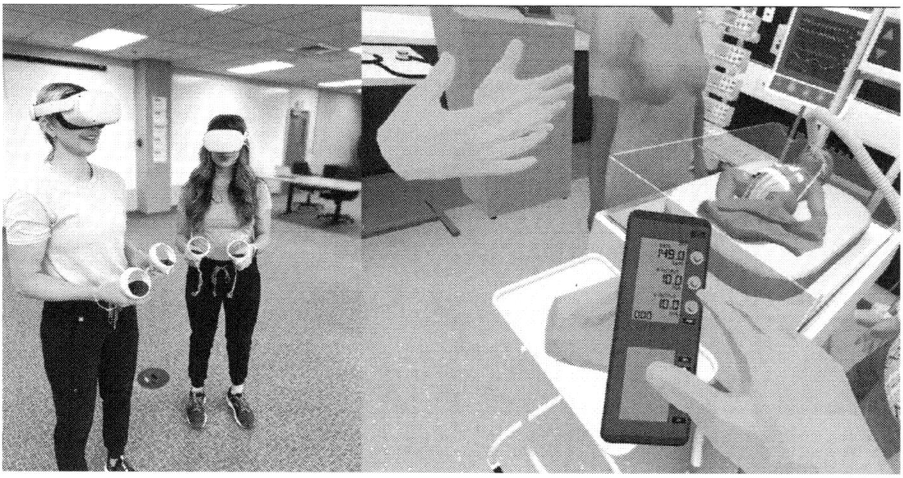

(Photo courtesy of SimX, used with permission)

Chapters 3-8 provided potential VR education and training solutions. By now, I'm sure you have already identified at least three to five other skills or topics where VR could make an impact. Write them down and start exploring the possibilities!

____

____

____

____

____

I am not suggesting that everyone should start a business to help address the inefficiencies of our healthcare system. But we all share a professional responsibility to do something about them. You can join internal committees, working groups, or associations or advance your education to add more innovation at your workplace.

Disclaimer: I have never taken business classes, so what I am about to suggest is strictly experiential and may conflict with what is taught in business school. If you have a business idea, consider the following steps as a basic roadmap.

1. **Figure out why your idea matters.** The first step toward developing a business is identifying the type of problem you want to solve. Will your idea make things more efficient? More effective? Will it benefit society? Or, maybe it's just your passion that brings you fulfillment. Either way, a business must fill an existing gap to eventually sustain itself. Do some market research: read the literature, speak with experts in the field, conduct polls on LinkedIn, etc. Most

importantly, leverage your own expertise to make the final determination.

2. **Start the business.** There are many different ways to start a business, but specific requirements and start-up costs are set forth by the state in which you are operating. You can seek help from a certified public accountant or even do it online through a reputable platform (I started mine through Incfile, which is now called Bizee). The filing process is what will make your business a legitimate company.

3. **Get educated.** I don't necessarily mean you should go to college to formally learn more about the services you plan to offer. What I mean is that you should learn as much as you can about what it is that you do. Become an expert. This will help you create a robust business plan that outlines your goals, how you will achieve them, and the timeframe in which you'd like to achieve them. This plan will likely be requested by investors and other prospective business partners. The basic components of a business plan include an executive summary, a company summary, a market analysis, a marketing plan, a team, and a financial summary.

4. **Build a network.** No matter how savvy you think you are, a business can only make it so far without a strong professional network. Always be prepared with an elevator pitch and be ready to engage with stakeholders. LinkedIn is a great platform for connecting with other professionals who share similar interests or may benefit from your services. Bundle of Rays (BoR) and XRenegades (a Firework Media company), are two great examples of VR subject-matter experts I discovered through LinkedIn. Founders Brad Chesham (BoR) and Tess McKinney (XRenegades) share my passion for

healthcare transformation and are already making an impact globally.

5. **Scale your idea.** Growing your business will require you to change your daily routine and consider strategies aimed at forming teams, establishing partnerships, investing in technology and marketing, outsourcing, and revising your business plan.

6. **Stick to evidence-based solutions.** The world around us evolves continuously, so staying on top of advances in our respective fields becomes critical. What worked five or ten years ago may no longer work today. Stay informed through newsletters, journals, webinars, and conferences.

This is what the process looked like when I started CLINSPEC Solutions, LLC.

1. Nursing shortages in the U.S. call for innovative solutions that promote cost-effective, safe, and reliable educational practices. Nursing simulations can be expensive and may not be readily accessible to all students. VR modalities are more affordable compared to high-fidelity simulators and are accessible to anyone who has a VR headset. VR in medical education is trending like never before, so why not provide implementation consultation services to organizations looking for a change?

2. As mentioned before, I founded CLINSPEC Solutions, LLC online. It was quick and easy! If your company is mainly owned by military veterans, it could also be eligible for veteran-owned business (VOB) certification. There are many benefits to VOB certification, so take the time to file this request through the Small Business Administration's website. Other certifications, such as woman-

owned, HUBZone, minority-owned, and small disadvantaged, are also worth exploring.

3. Enrolling in the Teaching and Learning in the Health Professions certificate program at MGH IHP was an excellent investment. Not only did it help fill many gaps in my knowledge, but it also led to an article publication in *STORM* [56] that advocates for the use of VR to educate and train vascular access specialists.

4. My professional network has grown exponentially since I founded CLINSPEC Solutions, LLC in 2023. I have leveraged LinkedIn and the MGH IHP student network and attended a few healthcare conferences to get the word out about VR education and training.

5. Just like the DoD depends on military-civilian partnerships to sustain clinical readiness, I, too, felt the need to establish symbiotic partnerships that synergize efforts to improve educational practices in healthcare. With BoR's learning management system (LMS), we can harness VR to reshape the way students and healthcare professionals learn and practice through 360° video, VR clinical simulation, metaverse platforms, soft skills capabilities, and VR anatomy. Most importantly, BoR can customize VR content to help meet the learning needs of the customer.

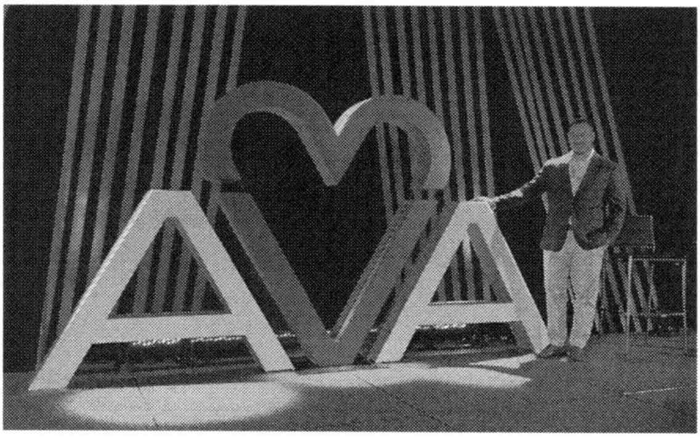

6. I subscribed to HealthySimulation.com, followed simulation education communities via LinkedIn, and became a member of the Association for Vascular Access to stay on top of the latest news.

Don't be that person who complains about everything but does nothing. As I have illustrated, there are many different ways to become more involved, both entrepreneurially and in other ways.

Regardless, innovative solutions like VR are revolutionizing the learning experience worldwide. With the assistance of VR implementation specialists like CLINSPEC Solutions and BoR, we can transform your traditional curriculum into an evidence-based VR curriculum that will take your performance to the next level.

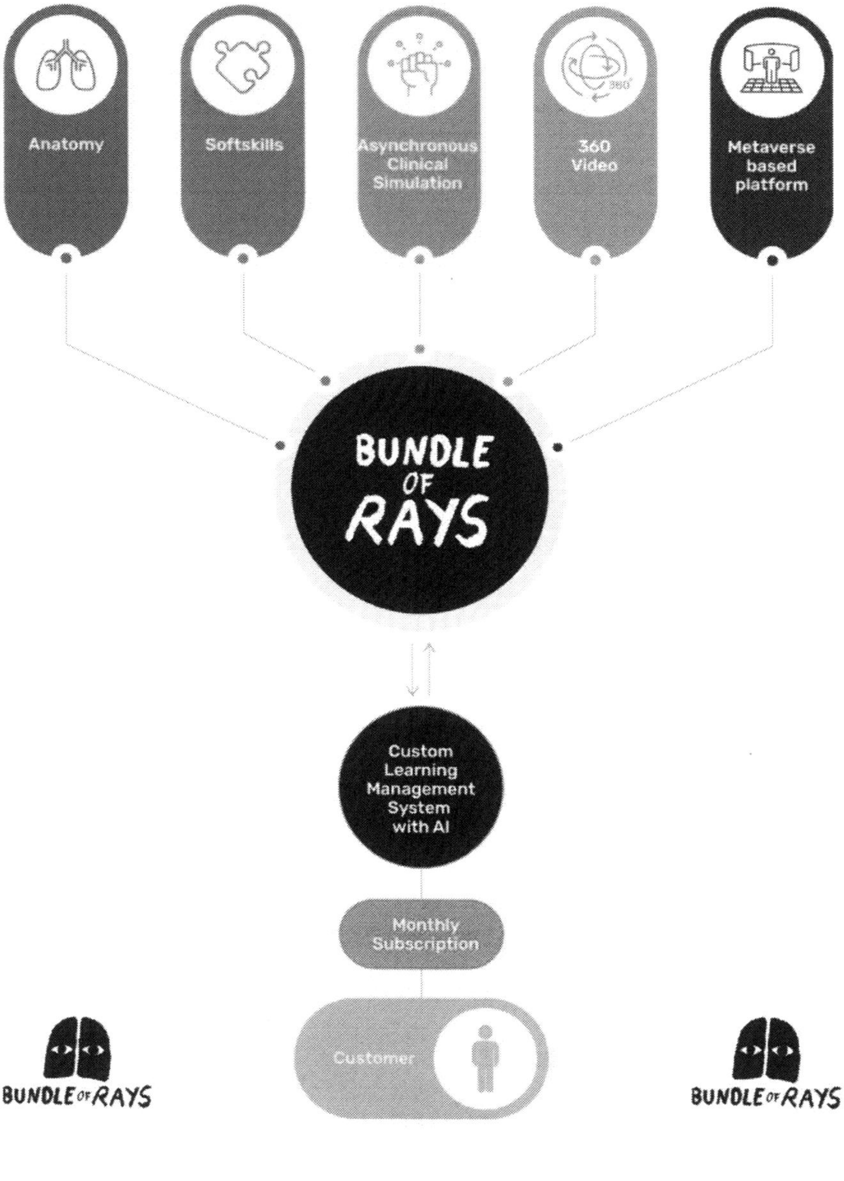

(Courtesy of Bundle of Rays, used with permission)

Conclusion

Now and then, I find myself reminiscing about life—especially now that I am retired from the military. What makes us who we are? I think we can all agree that we are a product of our life's journey: the good, the bad, and the ugly. We have journeyed through examples of my life experiences that have sparked innovative solutions in healthcare. Often, bad experiences ignite ideas—the type of ideas that make us ask how we can make things better in an ever-changing workforce. We will not keep pace with change if we don't learn to embrace innovative strategies.

I challenge you to reflect on your personal and professional experiences. New ideas come from the people and entities that have impacted you the most: patients like Mr. Norman Lafair, family members like Jose Pequeño and Nelida Bagley, mentors like HMCS Peter Espitia, BMCS Thomas Hatten, LT Tracy Isaac, LCDR Andrea Petrovanie, LCDR Carlin Calloway, LCDR Joseph Hacinas, LCDR David Crumbley, CDR Sarah Martin, CDR Dan Marino, CDR Candy Simmons, and CAPT Brenda Baker. They may come from leaders like William Bester and CAPT Jeffery Johnson, or business partners like PICC Pros, CVC Health Care, Precision Vascular Access, Peak Vascular Access, VATCO, and ComplyDash. Perhaps you had exemplary experiences with educators like Anne Muller, Ruth Lebet, Katie Davitt, and Suzie Kardong-Edgren or organizations like the U.S. Navy. Personally, my biggest supporters have been my family.

What will it cost to introduce immersive VR technology in healthcare education and training? The fact that medical errors are the third leading cause of death in the U.S. (about 795,000 deaths and injuries per year) is alarming. It is evident that traditional methods are insufficient and, in some cases, the problem is further compounded by high costs. When properly implemented, VR can offer a myriad of benefits to learners, educators, and, ultimately, patients (see the VR implementation checklist in Chapter 9). The use of VR can help standardize health curricula, offer helpful repetition when practicing complex procedures, make learning more accessible, and reduce training costs. In the case of PICC and midline insertion education and training, VR can aid the unstructured and disorganized characteristics of vascular access training programs. But it wasn't until I began connecting all the dots that I became aware of the applicability of VR in healthcare. Chapters 3 through 8 identified a handful of potential VR solutions in healthcare education and training (and one non-VR platform for compliance management), but the list goes on and can grow even longer with your input.

If you think you have an idea that could benefit the workplace, profession, or maybe even the world, don't be afraid to jump on the bandwagon and head into entrepreneurship. Give it a shot and see what happens. Perhaps it's a business idea someone else has already thought about and created. In that case, make it even better. If things were always done perfectly the first time, we would only have one brand of everything: vehicle, clothing, airline, laptop, cell phone, television, etc. But no, we have plenty to choose from. Starting a business is like writing a book; if you only focus on the end, you will most likely get burned out. So, take it one step at a time and have fun with the process.

Speaking of writing, John P. Roach Jr. inspired me to write a book long ago. Though we were separated by forty-five years of life, we met regularly at The Lion's Share in downtown San Diego in 2011 and 2012 (while I was stationed at NMCSD) to drink Duvel beer. He was a veteran, businessman, adventurer, musician, writer, and many more things. But I knew him as a world traveler who was inspired by his experiences. His book, *Essence of an Idealist*, depicts his story well: the ups and downs. His life was a roller coaster. This book follows in his footsteps and his hope that readers who read this memoir will find inspiration, too.

If you are an influencer in healthcare and looking for innovative solutions to old-school problems, shift your attention to VR. Credible VR platforms like BoR can customize learning content to fit your needs. But before you reach out, be diligent with planning out your initiatives: identify the problem, collect information related to the problem, perform a literature search, organize your findings, and evaluate your findings. For assistance with this process, consider connecting with a VR implementation consultant. CLINSPEC Solutions, LLC offers comprehensive support to guide organizations through every phase of their VR journey. From initial planning stages to seamless implementation, we collaborate with clients to tailor solutions so that they align with their unique goals and challenges. By leveraging cutting-edge technology and best practices, CLINSPEC Solutions, LLC empowers healthcare entities to harness VR's full potential for education, training, and patient care.

The last thing I will leave you with is to think about the *why*. Why do you do what you do? Do you do it for the money or because you love it? I find it hard to find satisfaction in doing work that I don't believe in. If what Notorious B.I.G. said about money is true ("Mo Money Mo Problems"), then I would prefer not to have the extra cash. Instead, I'd rather keep God in the center of it all.

In the Bible, Colossians 3:23-24 reads, "Whatever you do, work at it with all your heart, as working for the Lord, not for men, since you know that you will receive an inheritance from the Lord as a reward."

Rather than advocating for change for personal gain, do it for the greater good.

Honestly, I lost count of how many times junior sailors, both enlisted and officers, would ask me what they needed to do to get promoted and if they should take on additional tasks to make their evaluations or fitness reports stand out. My responses were always to find an opportunity to do something they would love doing and naturally shine and not to take on extra tasks for the sake of standing out. Doing things for the wrong reasons leads to job dissatisfaction and failure. I am not implying that we should not go out of our comfort zones every now and then, but when we do, we must do so for the right reasons.

Founding CLINSPEC Solutions, LLC is a perfect example. It was out of my comfort zone in so many ways, but my genuine interest in making a difference in healthcare has made every challenge well worth it. That being said, I look forward to serving the healthcare sector to proliferate the use of VR further —not because of the solid revenue potential but because my life story has proven that the world needs it. To close, I would like to share one of John P. Roach Jr.'s most memorable passages from *Essence of an Idealist.*

I have written a lot of books on cruise ships. Typically, I sit in the catbird seat early in the morning, surrounded by windows overlooking the vast ocean at the very bow of the ship. People tend to stop by and say hello. A man named Al Noullet from Dallas, TX, walked up, introduced himself, and started a conversation.

Al Noullet	Every day, you are always in the same seat. Why is that?
John	So people know where to find me.
Al Noullet	You seem to be always working on your computer.
John	I write books, and from this vantage point, it is the most perfect of places to be inspired.
Al Noullet	It sure is.
John	I am nearing the end of a 101-day trip recommended by my wife that started with a safari in Africa. The safari was something she always wanted to do.
Al Noullet	I see you here every day, and you are always alone. Where is your wife?

John	My wife, Deborah Johnson, passed away seventeen months ago.
Al Noullet	No, she didn't. She has been sitting right there next to you!

John passed away several years ago, but I know that he, too, was sitting right beside me in my garage at home as I wrote this book, just as Deborah was there for him when he shared his life story.

Thank you all for being part of my inspiration!

References

1. Buchman, S., & Henderson, D. (2019). Interprofessional empathy and communication competency development in healthcare professions' curriculum through immersive virtual reality experiences. *Journal of Interprofessional Education & Practice, 15*, 127-130.

2. Chang, Y. M., & Lai, C. L. (2021). Exploring the experiences of nursing students in using immersive virtual reality to learn nursing skills. *Nurse Education Today, 97*, 104670.

3. Choi, J., Thompson, C. E., Choi, J., Waddill, C. B., & Choi, S. (2022). Effectiveness of immersive virtual reality in nursing education: systematic review. *Nurse Educator, 47*(3), E57-E61.

4. Saab, M. M., Hegarty, J., Murphy, D., & Landers, M. (2021). Incorporating virtual reality in nurse education: a qualitative study of nursing students' perspectives. *Nurse Education Today, 105*, 105045.

5. Smith, P. C., & Hamilton, B. K. (2015). The effects of virtual reality simulation as a teaching strategy for skills preparation in nursing students. *Clinical Simulation in Nursing, 11*(1), 52-58.

6. Woon, A. P. N., Mok, W. Q., Chieng, Y. J. S., Zhang, H. M., Ramos, P., Mustadi, H. B., & Lau, Y. (2021). Effectiveness of virtual reality training in improving knowledge among nursing students: A systematic review, meta-analysis and meta-regression. *Nurse Education Today, 98*, 104655.

7. Efendi, D., Apriliyasari, R. W., Prihartami Massie, J. G. E., Wong, C. L., Natalia, R., Utomo, B., ... & Chen, K. H. (2023). The effect of virtual reality

on cognitive, affective, and psychomotor outcomes in nursing staffs: systematic review and meta-analysis. *BMC nursing, 22*(1), 170.

8. Niemeyer, M. (2018). Effective patient safety education for novice RNs: A systematic review. *J Nurs Educ Pract, 8*(3), 103-115.

9. Shorey, S., & Ng, E. D. (2021). The use of virtual reality simulation among nursing students and registered nurses: A systematic review. *Nurse Education Today, 98*, 104662.

10. Villman, N., & Anamthuruhtil Cheriyan, V. (2020). The future of virtual reality in simulation training for nurses at workplaces: A literature review.

11. Edwards, T. C., Patel, A., Szyszka, B., Coombs, A. W., Liddle, A. D., Kucheria, R., ... & Logishetty, K. (2021). Immersive virtual reality enables scrub nurses to acquire technical skills in complex revisions of total knee arthroplasty. *Archives of Orthopaedic and Trauma Surgery, 141*(12), 2313-2321.

12. Paschold, M., Huber, T., Maedge, S., Zeissig, S. R., Lang, H., & Kneist, W. (2017). Laparoscopic assistance by operating room nurses: Results of a virtual-reality study. *Nurse Education Today, 51*, 68-72.

13. Dean, S., Halpern, J., McAllister, M., & Lazenby, M. (2020). Nursing education, virtual reality and empathy? *Nursing Open, 7*(6), 2056-2059.

14. Papageorgiou, A., Leinweber, J., Böhm, K., Constantinou, C., Kolokotroni, O., Kapreli, E., ... & Papadopoullou, C. (2022). The development of an empathy curriculum (empathy in health) for healthcare students using VR technology. *Empathy-Advanced Research and Applications*, 143.

15. Curran, V., Xu, X., Simmons, K., Fleet, L., Coombs, H., Porter, R., ... & Nuttall, R. M. (2022). A phenomenological study of the use of 360° Virtual Reality (VR) video in pediatric and neonatal resuscitation training. *Health and Technology*, 1-9.

16. Farra, S., Hodgson, E., Miller, E. T., Timm, N., Brady, W., Gneuhs, M., ... & Bottomley, M. (2019). Effects of virtual reality simulation on worker emergency evacuation of neonates. *Disaster medicine and public health preparedness*, *13*(2), 301-308.

17. Yang, S. Y., & Oh, Y. H. (2022). The effects of neonatal resuscitation gamification program using immersive virtual reality: A quasi-experimental study. *Nurse Education Today*, *117*, 105464.

18. Yu, M., & Mann, J. S. (2021). Development of virtual reality simulation program for high-risk neonatal infection control education. *Clinical Simulation in Nursing*, *50*, 19-26.

19. Chae, D., Kim, J., Kim, K., Ryu, J., Asami, K., & Doorenbos, A. Z. (2023). An immersive virtual reality simulation for cross-cultural communication skills: Development and feasibility. *Clinical Simulation in Nursing*, *77*, 13-22.

20. Rahimi, M., Khodabandeh Shahraki, S., Fatehi, F., & Farokhzadian, J. (2023). A virtual training program for improving cultural competence among academic nurse educators. *BMC Medical Education*, *23*(1), 445.

21. Khoshnoodifar, M., Emadi, N., Mosalanejad, L., Maghsoodzadeh, S., & Shokrpour, N. (2024). A new practical approach using TeamSTEPPS strategies and tools:–an educational design. *BMC Medical Education*, *24*(1), 22.

22. Qiao, J., Xu, J., Li, L., & Ouyang, Y. Q. (2021). The integration of immersive virtual reality simulation in interprofessional education: A scoping review. *Nurse Education Today*, *98*, 104773.

23. Bailey, S. K., Brannick, M. T., Bowling, F., Reiner, C. C., Lyons, D., Llerena, L. E., & Okuda, Y. (2023). Comparing capabilities of simulation modalities for training combat casualty care: perspectives of combat medics. *Military medicine*, usad460.

24. Barrie, G., & MD, R. J. R. Implementation of a Proof-of-Concept Virtual Reality Medical Simulation Training Capability for USAF Pararescuemen.

25. Qin, L., You, Z., Liu, B., & Luo, C. (2024). Development of virtual reality training system for combat musculoskeletal trauma care. *SIMULATION*, 00375497241238025.

26. Salinas, D. (2017). Viscoelastic studies: effective tools for trauma and surgical resuscitation efforts. *AORN Journal*, *105*(4), 370-383.

27. Laspro, M., Groysman, L., Verzella, A. N., Kimberly, L. L., & Flores, R. L. (2023). The Use of Virtual Reality in Surgical Training: Implications for Education, Patient Safety, and Global Health Equity. *Surgeries*, *4*(4), 635-646.

28. Mao, R. Q., Lan, L., Kay, J., Lohre, R., Ayeni, O. R., & Goel, D. P. (2021). Immersive virtual reality for surgical training: a systematic review. *Journal of Surgical Research*, *268*, 40-58.

29. Ntakakis, G., Plomariti, C., Frantzidis, C., Antoniou, P. E., Bamidis, P. D., & Tsoulfas, G. (2023). Exploring the use of virtual reality in surgical education. *World journal of transplantation*, *13*(2), 36.

30. Portelli, M., Bianco, S. F., Bezzina, T., & Abela, J. E. (2020). Virtual reality training compared with apprenticeship training in laparoscopic surgery: a meta-analysis. *The Annals of the Royal College of Surgeons of England, 102*(9), 672-684.

31. Couperus, K., Young, S., Walsh, R., Kang, C., Skinner, C., Essendrop, R., ... & Gorbatkin, C. (2020). Immersive virtual reality medical simulation: autonomous trauma training simulator. *Cureus, 12*(5).

32. Gomez, B. G., Winstead, J., Lopata, J., & McMahon, R. (2023). Closing the Trauma and Critical Care Gap: A Paradigm Shift through Virtual Reality and Augmented Reality. *Medical Journal, US Army Medical Center of Excellence (MEDCoE).*

33. Lu, J., Leng, A., Zhou, Y., Zhou, W., Luo, J., Chen, X., & Qi, X. (2023). An innovative virtual reality training tool for the pre-hospital treatment of cranialmaxillofacial trauma. *Computer Assisted Surgery, 28*(1), 2189047.

34. Patel, D., Hawkins, J., Chehab, L. Z., Martin-Tuite, P., Feler, J., Tan, A., ... Sammann, A. (2020). Developing virtual reality trauma training experiences using 360-degree video: Tutorial. *Journal of Medical Internet Research*, 22(12), e22420.

35. Bruno, R. R., Wolff, G., Wernly, B., Masyuk, M., Piayda, K., Leaver, S., ... & Jung, C. (2022). Virtual and augmented reality in critical care medicine: the patient's, clinician's, and researcher's perspective. *Critical Care, 26*(1), 326.

36. Kanschik, D., Bruno, R. R., Wolff, G., Kelm, M., & Jung, C. (2023). Virtual and augmented reality in intensive care medicine: a systematic review. *Annals of Intensive Care, 13*(1), 81.

37. Ralston, B. H., Willett, R. C., Namperumal, S., Brown, N. M., Walsh, H., Muñoz, R. A., ... & Yurasek, G. (2021). Use of virtual reality for pediatric cardiac critical care simulation. *Cureus, 13*(6).

38. Marks, B., & Thomas, J. (2022). Adoption of virtual reality technology in higher education: An evaluation of five teaching semesters in a purpose-designed laboratory. *Education and Information Technologies, 27*(1), 1287-1305.

39. Singh, G., Mantri, A., Sharma, O., & Kaur, R. (2021). Virtual reality learning environment for enhancing electronics engineering laboratory experience. *Computer Applications in Engineering Education, 29*(1), 229-243.

40. Salinas, D., Sartain, B. J., Sullivan, J. F., Moore, C. B., & Hefley, J. (2021). Implementing ultrasound-guided peripheral intravenous practices on a multi-service unit. *Medsurg Nursing, 30*(3), 168-180.

41. Salinas, D., Johnson, S. C., Conrardy, J. A., Adams, T. L., & Brown, J. D. (2019). Sustaining nursing grand rounds through interdisciplinary teamwork and interorganizational partnership. *AJN The American Journal of Nursing, 119*(4), 41-48.

42. Andersen, N. L., Jensen, R. O., Posth, S., Laursen, C. B., Jørgensen, R., & Graumann, O. (2021). Teaching ultrasound-guided peripheral venous catheter placement through immersive virtual reality: An explorative pilot study. *Medicine, 100*(27), e26394.

43. Salinas, D. (2024). Virtual Reality: Emerging Technology in Vascular Access Education and Training. *STORM*, 3(1).

44. Savir, S., Khan, A. A., Yunus, R. A., Rehman, T. A., Saeed, S., Sohail, M., ... Matyal, R. (2023). Virtual reality: The future of invasive procedure training? *Journal of Cardiothoracic and Vascular Anesthesia.*

45. Mahajan, A. P., Inniss, D. A., Benedict, M. D., Dennis, A. A., Kantor, T., Salavitabar, A., ... & Cohen, M. S. (2022). International mixed reality immersive experience: approach via surgical grand rounds. *Journal of the American College of Surgeons, 234*(1), 25-31.

46. Mahajan, A. P., Inniss, D. A., Benedict, M. D., Dennis, A. A., Kantor, T., Kinross, J. M., & Cohen, M. S. (2021). The first international surgical grand rounds using immersive mixed reality headset devices. *Journal of the American College of Surgeons, 233*(5), S116.

47. Salavitabar, A., Popov, V., Nelson, J., Benedict, M. D., Inniss, D. A., Mahajan, A. P., ... & Sinou, N., Sinou, N., & Filippou, D. (2023). Virtual reality and augmented reality in anatomy education during COVID-19 pandemic. *Cureus, 15*(2).

48. Miltykh, I., Kafarov, E. S., Covantsev, S., Dadashev, A. S., Skarlis, A. A., & Zenin, O. K. (2023). A new dimension in medical education: Virtual reality in anatomy during COVID-19 pandemic. *Clinical Anatomy, 36*(7), 1007-1015.

49. Sinou, N., Sinou, N., & Filippou, D. (2023). Virtual reality and augmented reality in anatomy education during COVID-19 pandemic. *Cureus, 15*(2).

50. Cheng, A., Fijacko, N., Lockey, A., Greif, R., Abelairas-Gomez, C., Gosak, L., & Lin, Y. (2024). Use of augmented and virtual reality in resuscitation training: A systematic review. *Resuscitation Plus, 18*, 100643.

51. Wares, C., Ellington, E., Kitchen, A., Runyon, M., Pearson, D., Bullard, M., ... & Tarantino, H. (2024). Virtual Reality CPR Training Improves

Knowledge Acquisition of Critical Tasks. *Journal of Regional Medical Campuses, 7*(1).

52. Bednar, M., Dufek, P., Lochmannova, A., Simon, M., & Bures, M. (2023, September). Use of virtual reality for education and training of emergency rescue system for crisis situations. In *Proceedings of the 15th International Conference on Education Technology and Computers* (pp. 142-147).

53. Dib, N., Alattas, N., Fatima, A., Obaidat, H., & Ismail, H. (2023, August). EMT VR–A Gamified Emergency Response Training System Using Virtual Reality and Artificial Intelligence. In *2023 IEEE Smart World Congress (SWC)* (pp. 1-6). IEEE.

54. Kman, N. E., Price, A., Berezina-Blackburn, V., Patterson, J., Maicher, K., Way, D. P., ... & Danforth, D. (2023). First Responder Virtual Reality Simulator to train and assess emergency personnel for mass casualty response. *Journal of the American College of Emergency Physicians Open, 4*(1), e12903.

55. Vogt, P., Boer, R., de Boer, M., Prins, H., Smit, J., Tuinstra, D., ... & Paans, W. (2023, July). Designing and evaluating a Virtual Reality training for paramedics to practice triage in complex situations. In *International Conference on Human-Computer Interaction* (pp. 503-522). Cham: Springer Nature Switzerland.

56. Rodrigues, J., Ruivo, P., & Oliveira, T. (2014). Software as a Service Value and Firm Performance-a literature review synthesis in Small and Medium Enterprises. *Procedia Technology, 16*, 206-211.

57. Turetken, O., Elgammal, A., van den Heuvel, W. J., & Papazoglou, M. P. (2012). Capturing compliance requirements: A pattern-based approach. *IEEE software, 29*(3), 28-36.

THANK YOU FOR READING MY BOOK!

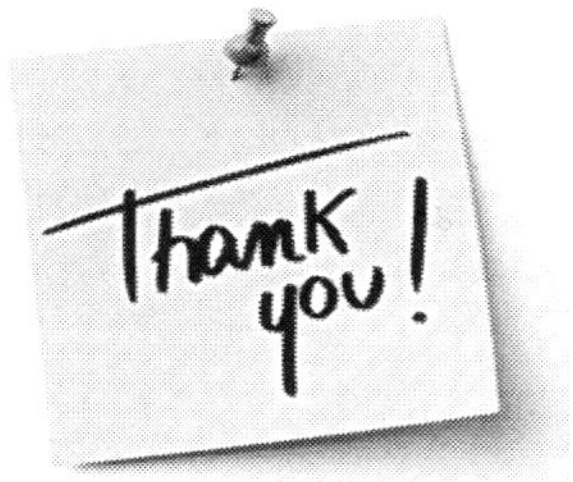

Discover the full range of services offered by CLINSPEC Solutions by scanning the QR code:

I appreciate your interest in my book and value your feedback as it helps me improve future versions of this book. I would appreciate it if you could leave your invaluable review on Amazon.com with your feedback. Thank you!